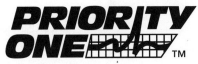

Emergency Preparedness and First Aid Guide

Priority One Publishing
Portland, Oregon

Published by Priority One Publishing,

PRIORITY ONE™

a division of Priority One Marketing International Inc.,
10647 S.W. River Drive, Portland, Oregon 97224

First published in 1994 by Priority One Publishing,
a division of Priority One Marketing International Inc.

Library of Congress Catalog Card Number: 93-87269

ISBN 0-96639782-0-9

Illustrations & cover design by Greg Milhem

Printed in the United States of America

1 2 3 4 5 6 7 8 9 10

To Gloria, Star, Samantha and Miranda

Acknowledgments

We would like to extend a special thank you to Oregon Health Sciences University, Department of Emergency Medicine for their outstanding support and contribution to the technical accuracy of this book. Their enthusiasm and willingness to participate in this project from the time it started, through its completion, is an affirmation of their excellent reputation in the field of emergency medicine.

Creating a book of this nature requires an abundance of time, hard work, patience, and care to turn out the very best product possible. In order to accomplish this, it also requires the cooperation of a dedicated team of professionals concerned with, and intimately familiar with, the subject matter. We have been extremely fortunate to have such a team of people involved in the creation of this book, all of whom, we are most gratefully thankful.

Oregon Health Sciences University
Department of Emergency Medicine
Portland, Oregon

Edward A. Bartkus - EMT-P, Assistant Professor
Mohamud R. Daya -MD, MS, FACEP, Assistant Professor
Jerris R. Hedges - MD, MS, FACEP, Professor
Jonathan Jui, MD - FACEP, Associate Professor
John C. Moorhead - MD, MS, FACEP, Professor: Chair, Department of Emergency Medicine
Martin J. Smilkstein - MD, FACEP, Assistant Professor
Eustacia (Jo) Su, MD - FACEP, Assistant Professor
Linda Tomassi - Department Manager, Emergency Medicine

City of Portland, Bureau of Fire, Rescue & Emergency Services
Portland, Oregon

Tony Anderegg - Staff Captain

Oregon Poison Center
Portland, Oregon

Sandra Giffin - Department Director

Washington County 911
Beaverton, **Oregon**
    Larry L. Hatch - Assistant Director

Central United States Earthquake Consortium
Memphis, Tennessee
    Andy Hellenthal - Mitigation Specialist

Doctors for Disaster Preparedness
Tucson, Arizona
    Howard Maccabee, M.D., Ph.D. - President

National Emergency Management Association
Washington, D.C.
    Roy C. Price, Sr. - Vice Director, Hawaii State Civil Defense
    Bill Norris - Population Protection Planner

National Fire Protection Association
Quincy, Massachusetts
    Numerous staff members

International Association of Fire Chiefs
Fairfax, Virginia
    Garry L. Briese, CAE - Executive Director

Emergency Nurses Association
Park Ridge, Illinois
    Eileen Corcoran, RN, BSN, CEN, MICN - 1993 President

City of Portland, Bureau of Police
Portland, Oregon
    Joe Midgett - Analyst, Statistical Support Unit
    Mary Otto - Crime Prevention Specialist

Insurance Agency
Tigard, Oregon
    Jim Miller - Agency Owner

Table of Contents

First Aid for Specific Injuries and Illnesses

Preface

The Priority One Emergency Preparedness and First Aid Guide brings together basic but important information that may some day help save your life, or the life of a friend or family member.

The guide is divided into two distinct sections: Emergency Preparedness and First Aid. The Emergency Preparedness section covers the important things you need to know and do in order to better survive both natural and man made emergency situations. The First Aid section covers first aid procedures for the most commonly occurring medical emergencies.

We highly recommend that you take the time to read the Emergency Preparedness section and at least the first 3 or 4 chapters in the First Aid section. These chapters provide information that's good to know before you're faced with any specific emergency situation.

The Priority One Emergency Preparedness and First Aid Guide was written with the assistance of some of the most knowledgeable professionals in the fields of emergency medicine and emergency preparedness. But despite the advanced knowledge that's behind the guide, it was written to be straightforward, interesting and easy to understand.

Now you have a guide that may help you through an emergency situation. And we hope that having this guide will help you rest a little easier.

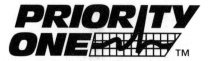

PRIORITY ONE ™

Emergency
Preparedness

Introduction

On Monday, March 22, 1993, at 5:35 in the morning, residents in the Pacific Northwestern United States woke to an earthquake. Houses shook, buildings swayed and the earth roared. Lasting up to 45 seconds and measuring 5.7 on the Richter scale, the tremor was felt from Southern Oregon to as far north as Seattle, Washington.

Ask anyone who woke to the quake that morning and they'll tell you it was the last thing they expected. In fact, if asked the day before, most people in the Pacific Northwest would have guessed that the next sizable quake would strike California, certainly not Oregon and Washington.

It Won't Happen to Me

This attitude is not uncommon. Most people feel that an emergency situation will not happen to them. Natural and man-made disasters happen to people in other states, in other parts of the country – certainly not in your city or neighborhood. And definitely not in your home. That's what the people of the Pacific Northwest thought prior to being awakened by an earthquake. But they don't think that any longer.

Learning from History

No one expected Hurricane Andrew to slam into South Florida and the Louisiana coast on August 24th through 26th, 1992, killing 14 people and causing possibly as much as $20 billion in damage. No one expected an earthquake measuring 7.8 on the Richter scale to strike in China on July 28, 1976, taking the lives of over 500,000 people. And no one expected that Johnstown, Pennsylvania, the site of the great 1889 flood which took 2,209 lives, would see history repeated in the 1977 flood which claimed 77 lives, 500 homes and caused $200 million in damage. And on a smaller scale, but equally as real, no one expects their home to catch fire during the night while they're sleeping.

And that's the point. There are certain things that are beyond our control so we simply choose not to think about them. Natural disasters create life-threatening emergency situations. They're a reality, but we treat them as if they're a long shot and ignore them. At least until we are forced to look them in the eye.

But as a society we're beginning to realize that the odds of encountering emergency situations are higher than we once thought. We're buying automobiles that have air bags, requiring children to ride in child-safety seats, wearing helmets when we ride bicycles, and there are more smoke detectors in more homes today than there were a year ago. We're waking up to the fact that dangers exist, and we're taking precautions. And precautions, or preparedness, is the key to survival.

There's Nothing Pessimistic about Preparedness

Thinking about and getting ready for potential emergency situations doesn't mean you have to live your life dwelling on them. Just the opposite is true really, because thinking about and planning for emergency situations now means you can alleviate subconscious anxiety you may have about being unprepared.

The Biggest Hurdle

"Preparedness takes too much time and there's too much to read." Most people think it takes too much time to make themselves prepared. But in fact, time and energy aren't the biggest hurdles to becoming prepared. It takes very little time and it's not complicated at all. Preparedness is mostly common sense information and a little organization. It's really easy. The biggest hurdle to becoming prepared then, is admitting that you need to. Ask anyone who's ever experienced an emergency situation and they'll tell you that if they would have been more prepared it would have made all the difference.

It Only Takes a Little Time

The emergency preparedness section of this book, as well as the first aid section, is meant to be easy to read and simple to understand. It truly is common sense information. At the very least, read the first few chapters of this section and spend a few hours putting together your survival supplies. That's the minimum. And if you do only that, you'll be prepared for almost any emergency situation.

We recommend, however, that you read the basics in each chapter and prepare yourself for all of the possible situations you may encounter. And reread chapters from time to time to refresh your memory. You'll be done after only spending a few hours of your time – a few hours that may save your life.

Before an Emergency

Emergencies can occur at any time, in any place. But even though you can't prevent most emergencies from happening (especially natural disasters) you can prepare for them.

The biggest part of preparation is assembling survival supplies, which are outlined in detail in the following section. You should also become familiar with the location of your local emergency shelter. But in addition to these physical things, you can also help ensure your survival by mentally preparing for emergency situations.

Talk About it Before it Happens

Talk to your family, especially children, about what it would be like to experience an emergency situation. Talk about household fires and any specific natural disaster your community may be susceptible to and develop a family disaster plan. Becoming familiar with potential emotions like loss and loss of control, and understanding that there's a lot you can do together as a team, will begin to lessen their fears when you're faced with an emergency situation.

Keeping Calm can Keep you Safe

Imagine too, how you would act when faced with an emergency situation. Try now to prepare yourself mentally for such situations. Because moods can be very contagious, especially in high-stress situations, it's always best that you remember to remain calm and controlled. Those around you will sense your mood and will also remain calm. A stable emotional state leads to more sound thinking. And sound thinking in the face of an emergency can mean the difference between life and death.

Survival Supplies

Everyone has, at one time or another, been in a situation where they didn't plan ahead. Most of the time this lack of planning isn't very serious. It may be something as simple as forgetting to buy a certain ingredient for a recipe. Most of the time this lack of planning results in an inconvenience that can be taken care of quickly with no real discomfort involved.

But not planning ahead for an emergency situation will not only be inconvenient, it may be life-threatening. That's why planning ahead for emergencies can make all the difference in the world. Having the right survival supplies on hand is a very big and very important part of emergency preparedness. The survival supplies on the following pages will be continually referred to throughout this book. It's very important that you become familiar with the survival supplies you need, and that you gather them. Because unlike an ingredient for a recipe, when you need survival supplies you can't just run out to a convenience store and buy them.

If you don't have them soon, chances are you won't have them when you really need them – during an emergency.

It seems that no matter what type of emergency situation you're faced with, the supplies you'll need vary only slightly. That's why our list is a multi-purpose list, serving your survival needs for just about any emergency situation – from an earthquake or a flood, to a fire or a power outage.

How to Store your Supplies

Keep items in air tight plastic bags such as "Zip Lock®" bags. Keep items you would most likely need in the event of an evacuation in an easy to carry container. Suggestions include: a camping backpack, a duffel bag, or a large, covered trash container.

Where to Store your Survival Supplies

Keep your survival supplies out of the way but not hidden away. An area in your basement or in a closet would do. The area you choose should be clean, dry and used exclusively for survival supplies. There will be certain supplies that need to be rotated out every six months, so be sure that your storage area is accessible on a daily basis. It's also important to keep your supplies neat and organized so when it comes time to use them you won't waste any time locating anything. And make sure all family members know where these supplies are kept.

Medical Supplies

In addition to your first aid kit and this book, you should include any personal medication and perhaps extra pairs of prescription eye glasses. Be sure to rotate out any prescription medications. Ask your physician or pharmacist about storing prescription medications.

The following pages contain check lists to help you organize your survival supplies. The lists are extensive. You may have to edit them according to your personal resources and storage space restrictions. Start with the essentials like water, food and clothing, then see what you can add.

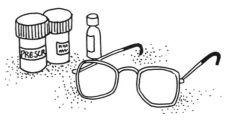

Clothing

A clean change of warm clothing for each member of your family should be among your supplies. Remember, rugged clothes are best, since you may need as much protection as you can get during an emergency.

Clothing items for each member of your family should at least include:

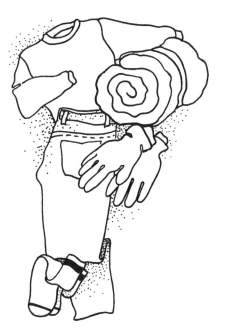

- ☐ Shirts
- ☐ Jackets
- ☐ Pants
- ☐ Underwear
- ☐ Socks

- ☐ Sturdy shoes or boots
- ☐ Hats
- ☐ Warm, heavy gloves
- ☐ Scarves
- ☐ Warm, heavy blankets/ sleeping bags

Food, Water and Supplies

A supply of food and water to last at least three days to as long as seven days is a vital part of your survival supplies. Rotate your emergency food and water supplies into your everyday supplies every six months, and replace your emergency supplies with a fresh stock.

- ☐ Canned fruit
- ☐ Canned vegetables
- ☐ Canned meat
- ☐ Canned fish
- ☐ Rice
- ☐ Canned soup
- ☐ Pasta
- ☐ Cereal
- ☐ Bread
  (store in freezer)

- ☐ Canned or powdered milk
- ☐ Canned or bottled beverages
- ☐ Snacks
- ☐ One gallon of water per person, per day
- ☐ Manual can opener
- ☐ Outdoor cooking stove
- ☐ Pots and pans

Commercially sealed multi-gallon containers of water are the easiest to deal with. And non-perishable, canned and dehydrated food that doesn't necessarily need to be heated is recommended. Suggestions for assembling your "survival pantry" include:

- ☐ Cooking fuel/Sterno
- ☐ Eating utensils
- ☐ Paper plates
- ☐ Cups
- ☐ Paper towels
- ☐ Garbage container
- ☐ Plastic garbage bags and ties
- ☐ Aluminum foil
- ☐ Liquid detergent

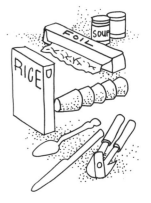

Hygiene

Keeping clean is important, especially during a disaster since dirt and germs may be more prevalent.

☐ Antibacterial soap, liquid detergent
☐ Personal hygiene items
☐ Wash and dry towelettes
☐ Kleenex
☐ Towels
☐ Household bleach for disinfection
☐ Toilet paper
☐ Portable toilet or sturdy bucket with lid
☐ Plastic bags and ties to serve as portable toilet liners
☐ Feminine supplies

Tools

Because you never know how serious household damage can be, a good supply of emergency tools is recommended.

☐ Shovel
☐ Axe
☐ Broom and dust pan
☐ Strong rope, at least 50 ft.
☐ Fire extinguisher
☐ Utility knife, pocket knife
☐ Razor blades
☐ Wrench
☐ Pliers
☐ Screw drivers

☐ Hammer
☐ Nails
☐ Plywood
☐ Staple gun
☐ Strong tape
☐ Tools necessary to turn off gas and water utilities
☐ Plastic sheeting

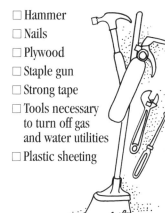

Miscellaneous

There are many items that don't fit into a category that are simply smart things to include with your survival supplies.

- ☐ Battery powered radio
- ☐ Extra set of car keys
- ☐ Money/change/ travelers checks
- ☐ Clock or wrist watch
- ☐ Escape ladder
- ☐ Flashlights/lanterns
- ☐ Candles/light sticks
- ☐ Matches
- ☐ Paper and pencil or pen

- ☐ Tent
- ☐ Pet food
- ☐ Activity books for children
- ☐ Deck of cards
- ☐ Toys and games for children
- ☐ Whistle

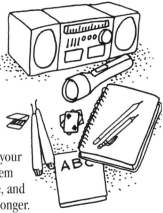

To avoid battery corrosion inside a clock or flashlight, it's important that you keep batteries out of the devices until you need to use them. Storing batteries in your freezer will keep them out of every day use, and will help them last longer.

Think about any other items that may be unique to your family or family members. Are there special considerations (formula, food, medications etc.) you need to make for an infant? And elderly person? A disabled person?

Survival Supplies for Your Automobile

It's smart to keep survival supplies in the trunk of your car for emergencies. Your supplies should include:

- ☐ Road flares
- ☐ Rain gear
- ☐ Warm clothes
- ☐ Hat and gloves
- ☐ Walking shoes
- ☐ Flashlight
- ☐ Battery powered radio
- ☐ Batteries
- ☐ Water

- ☐ Food
- ☐ Maps
- ☐ Shovel
- ☐ Sand
- ☐ Ice scraper/brush

- ☐ First aid kit
- ☐ Compass
- ☐ Booster cables
- ☐ Matches
- ☐ Blankets/sleeping bags

Disaster Insurance

There are a variety of disaster insurance policies available. The cost of a policy generally depends upon the specific disaster you're insuring against, the likelihood of the disaster occurring in your area, how comprehensive the policy is, the value of your home or the belongings you're insuring, and the insurance company itself.

Considering that Hurricane Andrew caused over $900 million in personal property damage when it struck South Florida in 1992, and considering that over $400 million of that was uninsured damage, the need for disaster insurance becomes very real.

Disaster insurance is usually dictated by one's personal economic situation, but if you're fortunate enough to have disaster insurance or if you're thinking about getting a policy, there are a few things you may want to consider.

Choosing your Policy

The first thing you need to do is decide what type of disaster you would like to insure against. No matter where you live, your home or apartment is susceptible to theft and fire. So theft and fire insurance should be on your list. Then you need to consider where you live. Is your particular area prone to tornados? Does your area have a history of flooding? What about hurricanes? And how susceptible is your city or state to earthquakes? Remember, California isn't the only state with a history of earthquakes. Earthquakes occur in the majority of America's states.

Once you decide on the disasters your area is more prone to experience, you can start investigating policies that can protect you and your belongings. Get several quotes from established insurance companies. Compare the premiums with the extent of the coverage. Don't forget to factor in the deductible if there is one. And once you decide on your policy, you'll find that it not only protects your home or belongings, but it provides peace-of-mind as well.

Pre-Documentation

Because insurance protects the value of what you chose to insure, it's important that you have some proof or a record of its value before any disaster occurs. If you insure your home and its contents, for example, it's wise to document everything that's covered by your policy with the use of still photography or a video camera. Also, a property profile form which may serve as a record of your valuables, is located at the back of this book. Be sure to take time to complete the forms.

Photographing anything and everything that's covered by your policy will not only provide proof of your possessions, but will also serve to speed up your refund. Remember to store the photographs or the video tape, and your insurance policy, in a safe place. Storing your documentation in a fireproof safe, safety deposit box or somewhere off premises like at a friend's house or at your place of work is a good idea. You wouldn't want the proof of your possessions to go up in flames along with possessions.

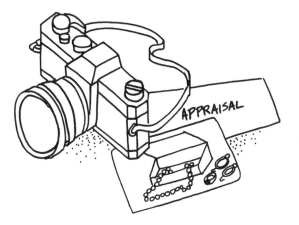

In most cases a visual representation is enough. However, the specific value of some things, like jewelry or diamonds for example, can't be determined by photography alone. Diamonds, jewelry, antiques, collectibles etc., need to be appraised by a professional, certified appraiser in order to protect their value. Also, some of these things are not covered by regular policies. It's important that you let your insurance company know of any unusual items of value you have in case they require special policies of their own.

Post-Documentation

If your house burns down, it's obvious what you have lost. But if your house has suffered flood or earthquake damage, for example, your losses are not as obvious. That's why it's important to document the damage, again, with still photography or video tape, immediately after the damage occurs. And because people have an instinct to "clean up" after a disaster, post-documentation should be done before you clean up.

And remember, if your home is unsafe to be in, don't even bother to document any damage. Your insurance appraiser will take care of it safely. Your possessions are not worth risking your life.

Earthquakes

Earthquakes have taken millions of lives over the centuries. And as recently as 1976, serious earthquakes have struck China, Guatemala, Indonesia, the Philippines, Turkey and Northern Italy claiming as many as 700,000 lives that year alone. Considering that earthquakes have struck at varying intensities in the majority of America's states, earthquake preparedness is not only smart, it's vital to survival.

Many people, even in states more susceptible to earthquakes like California, tend to ignore the fact that earthquakes can and will strike. No one likes to think about a potential disaster. But not thinking about it and not preparing for it now, could mean you may not be alive to think about it in the future. It's that simple.

Earthquakes are a reality, and there's a lot you can do to lessen potential damage and suffering. Even the basics will help increase your chances of surviving.

Before an Earthquake

Safety Zones

Every room in every home has a safety zone. The central area of a house or building is usually the sturdiest. That means the inside corner of a room away from windows or an inner wall make good safety zones. Even a heavy table or desk that you can crawl under and hold on to is good. Study your home carefully and determine the safety zone in each room. Then practice locating each zone with all family members.

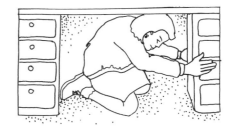

Meeting Place

Determine a place where all family members will meet after an earthquake.

Damage Prevention

Some damage caused by earthquakes is preventable. Especially the loss or damage to dishware, bookshelves, pictures, mirrors – anything that's breakable and not normally secured. Just add extra stability and security to the things that are breakable. Latches or bolts on cabinet doors will prevent the cabinets from opening and their contents from falling out during a quake. Also, securing large, heavy furniture items (like mirrors and picture frames) to walls can prevent potential damage. Water heaters are also vulnerable during an earthquake. Consider adding straps to prevent major appliances and storage tanks from shifting and breaking. Making sure your water heater and other appliances are extra secure may someday be appreciated.

Long-Distance Contact

Local telephone service may be out of order for days after a quake strikes, but in many states long distance service has a tendency to remain operating. For this reason, establishing a long-distance contact, an out-of-state family or friend, may be your best method for keeping in touch with family members in other parts of your city or state. Just make sure that everyone you want to be in contact with has the number of your long-distance contact. **(See Important Telephone Numbers at the back of this book.)**

Plan with your Neighbors

Develop a plan of action with your neighbors. How can you help each other? How can you work together to survive for at least 72 hours without government assistance? Share your discoveries and plans with non-neighbors like other friends and relatives.

During an Earthquake

- Try to remain calm.

- When the shaking starts and you're inside your house or apartment, head to the nearest safety zone. Stay clear of anything that may fall or break like bookshelves, dishes, windows and glass doors.

- If you're unable to reach a safety zone, cover yourself with anything (blankets, towels etc.) that gives at least some protection from falling objects or breaking glass.

- If in a building during and earthquake many people instinctively want to get out. You should never evacuate a building while the earth is still moving. If you're indoors, take cover immediately. Do not evacuate the building until the shaking has stopped and you have made a quick visual inspection (60 seconds) for hazards. Also, check yourself for injuries.

When you do evacuate the building, watch for any overhead objects like parts of the building or power lines that could cause injuries.

- If you're already outside when a quake strikes, stay outside. Move to an open area away from things that may fall like power lines, buildings and trees. And if you happen to see downed power lines, stay away from them **(see "Look out for power lines" at the end of this chapter).**

- If you're driving in your car as a quake begins, drive to the nearest open area and stop. Stay in your car until the shaking stops. When you begin driving, be cautious – there may be cracks in streets and power lines down.

Immediately Following an Earthquake

- Remain calm. Stay where you are until you think the earthquake has ended. Expect after shocks. As many as 40 to 60 can occur per hour immediately after an earthquake.

- Leave your safety zone cautiously only after you're sure the initial quake has ended.

- Administer emergency first aid procedures as necessary. See your Priority One First Aid Guide for information on specific injuries.

- Don't turn on lights or create sparks or flames. There may be a gas leak.

- If you smell or hear leaking gas, turn your gas off at the meter, **(see illustration 1)** open windows and call your gas company for further instructions. Don't attempt to turn the gas on before the gas company

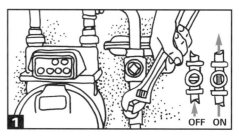

has checked out your gas lines and has determined that they are safe.

- Try to access your emergency supplies. Protect yourself by putting on your heavy clothes and sturdy shoes.

- Tune in to local emergency information on your battery powered radio. Evacuate only if you are told to do so.

- Cautiously check your home for structural damage. Check your chimney for cracks. Chimneys are susceptible to damage and could fall in the hours after the earthquake.

- Check your telephone to see that the quake hasn't shaken the receiver from its cradle. Also, limit your telephone use to emergency calls only.

- Be on the lookout for fire hazards. Check your appliances. If they're smoking or sparking, or you notice any damage to service outlets, disconnect your electricity by switching off your main breaker. In an older house, pull your fuse cartridge from its socket.

- If you feel your home or building is unsafe to remain in, go to your nearest local emergency shelter. Take your emergency supply kit with you (remember, it has the medications and other personal items you may need). Expect to be at the shelter for 72 hours or more.

During the Hours After an Earthquake

- Don't drive anywhere unless absolutely necessary.

- Take photos of household damage for insurance purposes before you begin cleaning up.

- Carefully clean up any broken glass or any other potentially dangerous damage.

- Before you flush toilets, make sure your sewage lines are not broken.

- Open closets and cupboards carefully, so as not to be struck by their contents.

- Notify your family contact. Let them know how you and your family are doing, so that they can assure worried relatives. Otherwise, use your telephone for emergencies only.

- Remember to eat as well as you can and to drink fluids. Eat foods in refrigerator first, then eat from the freezer. Eat canned foods last.

- Stay away from coastal areas where Tsunamis (earthquake induced tidal waves) may strike.

- Evacuate only if told to do so. Listen to your battery powered radio to learn if you need to evacuate. Emergency personnel will give evacuation route information.

- If you do evacuate and only if time permits, shut off your electricity, gas and water lines before leaving your home.

- Leave a note on your front door identifying where you will be and your evacuation route in case others are concerned or looking for you.

Look Out for Power Lines

Typically, as a result of an earthquake electrical power lines fall. And because your body, as well as metal and just about any moist or wet object, is a good conductor of electricity, coming in contact with downed power lines can cause serious injury or even death. For this reason it's best to look out for and stay away from downed power lines.

If live power lines come in contact with your car and you're in it, stay inside your car until professional rescuers arrive. Most cars are insulated, providing protection from electricity as long as you avoid contact with metal parts of the car. Similarly, avoid rescuing anyone from a car with downed power lines contacting it.

Extreme Temperatures

Just like an earthquake or tornado can damage your surroundings, any extreme fluctuation in the temperature of your environment can damage your body, and can even kill you. In fact, thousands of people die each year from extreme temperatures.

Because this chapter deals more with the human body than others in the Emergency Preparedness section, it's important that you use this chapter in conjunction with the chapters on Cold Exposure and Heat Illness in the Priority One First Aid section.

Heat

What is Heat Illness?

The human body can withstand much greater decreases in temperature than it can increases in temperature. And because of this, more people die each year from extreme heat than do people from extreme cold or hypothermia.

When the body's temperature rises, its natural reaction is to cool itself through sweating. Too much sweating can cause dehydration as well as a loss of salt, which your body needs. If lost water and salt are not replaced quickly, one may suffer from heat exhaustion. Heat exhaustion is a more mild form of heat stroke. Its symptoms include sweating, cool skin, dilated pupils, headache, thirst, nausea, vomiting, dizziness and weakness.

Symptoms of heat stroke include dry skin (not sweaty) that is hot and red, contracted pupils, a rapid but weak pulse, rapid and shallow breathing, confusion, weakness, seizures and unconsciousness.

Who does Heat Illness Effect?

Typically, warm climates as well as more temperate climates can experience rather sudden, extreme and prolonged rises in temperature, otherwise known as heat waves. Infants, young children, the elderly and those in poor health are more susceptible to heat illness than others. If members of your family fall into any of these groups, it's important that you watch them carefully for symptoms of heat illness during heat waves. But they're not alone. Everyone is susceptible to heat illness. Young, healthy adults, especially when exercising or working hard in unusually warm temperatures, may be overcome by heat.

How do you Prevent Heat Illness?

Your natural reaction to keep cool during a heat wave is absolutely correct. Wearing loose, light clothing; taking cool showers; applying cool compresses; taking advantage of air conditioned environments; using electric fans and keeping your physical activities to a minimum all help your body stay cool.

How do you Treat Heat Illness?

The "cure" for heat exhaustion is very similar to its preventive measures – keep cool. The first thing is to get the victim out of the warm environment and into a cool one. Cool compresses, lightly salted drinks and the removal of warm clothing will all help the victim cool down. Heat stroke requires similar measures, with the addition of medical attention being sought immediately.

(For more detailed information about first aid measures for heat exhaustion and heat stroke, see the Heat Illness chapter in the Priority One First Aid Section.)

Cold

What is Hypothermia?

Hypothermia occurs when the body's temperature drops dramatically. Symptoms of mild hypothermia include shivering, an urge to urinate, loss of coordination and confusion. Severe hypothermia victims are usually no longer shivering, they may experience weakness, muscle stiffness and an irregular or slow heartbeat. In many cases, frostbite accompanies hypothermia.

Who does Hypothermia Effect?

Just like heat illness, hypothermia strikes just about anyone, anywhere. Certain people, however, are more prone to hypothermia than others. They include infants, young children, the elderly and those in poor health. If members of your family fall into any of these groups, it's important that you watch them carefully for signs of hypothermia, especially after being in a cold environment for an extended period of time.

How do you Prevent Hypothermia?

Keep warm. It's that simple. Do everything you can to keep yourself or someone else from becoming cold. And that means if the heat in your house is not working and it's cold outside, leave your house and go to someplace warm. In the event of emergencies, your local Red Cross chapter may be able to refer you to a warming center. Also, you may want to have an emergency generator in your home to power your furnace, electrical appliances and lights. But consult your local gas or electric company first.

How do you Treat Hypothermia?

Seek medical help immediately. There are some things you can do while waiting for medical help to arrive. First, get the victim into warm, dry clothing and cover the victim with heavy blankets and quilts. If necessary, warm the victim with your own body. Apply warm compresses to the victim's neck, chest and groin area. And if the victim is awake, alert and can swallow, give warm, sweetened liquids or soup.

(For more detailed information about first aid measures for hypothermia, see the Cold Exposure chapter in the Priority One First Aid Section.)

Flooding

Thousands of people die worldwide each year from flooding. In the United States an annual average of $1 billion in property damage results from flooding, and as many as 200 people die from flood waters. During the summer of 1993 alone, the Midwestern United States suffered at least $10 billion in damage throughout 9 states.

Like other powerful acts of nature, flooding is something we have very little control over. Dams, dikes, and drainage systems work to a degree, but nature inevitably runs its course.

Before a Flood

Choosing your Home

If you're in the position to buy a home, or are planning on building a new home, one factor in your selection process is location. Location consists of neighborhood, schools, taxes and the like. But location should also consist of the immediate terrain, including the potential for flooding. Buying or building a home on or adjacent to a flood plain or flood prone area obviously exposes your home and your life to the potential dangers of flooding. Even elaborate levy systems, as demonstrated by the Midwest floods of 1993, are not completely effective in preventing floods.

Today, as many as 15 million Americans live in the path of potential flood waters. Most of these homes were built before today's tighter regulations and building codes were in place. So what can these people do to help lessen the danger and damage of flooding?

Flood Insurance

Flood insurance, like any disaster insurance, can make all the difference in the world. Flood insurance may be purchased to protect the belongings of renters as well. Contact your insurance agent to learn more about the coverage available in your area **(see Disaster Insurance page 14 and the Property Profile forms at the back of this book).**

Survival Supplies

In addition to the survival supplies listed in the Survival Supplies section on **page 7,** you may want to include sandbags if you have the available space. Also, try to store your primary survival supplies above potential flood waters, like in a second floor closet or attic.

Evacuation Plan

Develop a family evacuation plan. Where will you go? What is the the nearest place, above potential flood waters, that you could reach safely? What is the safest route to your destination? Remember, low-lying roads and bridges may be impassable. Be sure to tell family and friends now about your evacuation plan so you won't have to worry about telling them when the time comes to actually evacuate.

If you do evacuate, leave a note on your front door identifying where you will be and your evacuation route in case others are concerned or looking for you.

During a Flood

- Stay tuned to local emergency weather information. In most cases advanced flood warning is provided. If a flood warning is issued for your area, flooding is occurring or will occur soon. Evacuate if you are told to do so.

- If evacuation is necessary and if time permits, turn off all electric utilities at the main switch. Don't touch electrical equipment if it or you are exposed to water.

- If time permits, open basement windows to help equalize water pressure on walls and foundations.

- Avoid areas that are already flooded. Remember, flood waters are deceptive and may be much deeper than you think. Don't cross any flooded areas on foot if the water is above your knees.

- Don't drive on flooded roads. Roads that are covered with flood waters are extremely dangerous. If you evacuate in your car at night, be extra alert for flood waters.

- If you are in your home when flood waters rise, go to your second floor or roof. Take your survival supplies with you and wait to be rescued. Don't attempt to swim to dry ground.

- Flash floods happen quickly and in many cases there is no warning. If a flash flood is taking place or if your area is issued a flash flood warning, you should seek higher ground immediately. If you're driving, avoid low-lying areas like ditches, creeks and rivers.

After a Flood

- Contact you insurance agent and have your policy and your Property Profile forms ready.

- Before you re-enter your house, be sure that it is structurally safe.

- Don't light a match or bring a candle or other flame into your house. There may be explosive gasses present.

- Be sure your electricity is turned off, and don't use any lights or appliances until an electrician has inspected your electrical system to be sure it is safe.

- For insurance purposes, take photographs of the damage before you begin cleaning up.

- Open windows to help dry out and air out your house.

- To minimize structural damage, pump out one third of the water in your basement each day.

- Always be aware of downed power lines and avoid them.

Fires

Nearly 4,000 people die each year in home and other building fires, and tens of thousands of people are injured. Today, as more and more homes are equipped with smoke detectors, and as building codes are enforced more strictly, the devastation from fires is less than what it was years ago. But today there are also more people and more homes, which means more exposure to fires.

Preventing a fire from starting in the first place, and knowing what to do if and when you're faced with a fire, will greatly improve your odds for survival. From installing smoke detectors to being on the lookout for potential fire hazards, there's nothing complicated about fire safety. It's common sense and it's simple. And it may simply save your life.

Fire Safety

Smoke Detectors Save Lives

- Install at least one smoke detector on each level of your home, including one outside each sleeping area.

- Smoke detectors should be installed high on a wall or ceiling but not near heat registers or doors and windows.

- If you install a smoke detector on a wall, it should be within 12 inches from the ceiling, but not closer than six inches.

- Install only smoke detectors that are approved by a testing and certification laboratory.

- Test your smoke detectors every month. Make it part of your routine, like taking out the trash or watering plants. It's a good idea to mark it on your calendar.

- If your smoke detector "chirps" it's most likely telling you the battery needs to be replaced. Replace batteries at least once a year and when detector "chirps".

- Immediately replace your smoke detectors if they are not working.

- Clean your smoke detector at least once a year since dust build-up is not good for smoke detectors.

- Never disconnect a smoke detector. If it sounds periodically from cooking or other non-fire causes, relocate it.

- Always keep fresh batteries on hand.

- Make sure everyone in your family knows what the smoke detector's alarm sounds like and how to respond.

Fire Extinguishers

- Fires should only be fought if the fire department has been called and everyone else is out of the building.

- If when fighting a fire the flames don't immediately die down, abandon the fire and escape.

- Every home should have at least one fire extinguisher and adult family members should know where it's located and how to use it.

- You may want to consider having additional fire extinguishers for the garage, workroom, etc..

- Store your fire extinguisher near a door where you can easily escape if necessary. Recommended areas include your kitchen, garage and near your furnace.

- Read the instructions for use and "recharging" that come with your specific fire extinguisher.

- Letters on the extinguisher indicate the class of fuel on which the fire extinguisher will be effective. "A" in a green triangle is for ordinary combustibles, "B" in a red square is for flammable liquids, "C" in a blue circle is for electrical equipment, and "C" in a yellow star is for combustible metals. "A" and "B" are most commonly used for household fires.

Look Out for Home Fire Hazards

- Be careful using cigarettes. Careless disposal of smoking materials is the number one cause of household fires.

- Don't smoke in bed when drowsy or medicated.

- If you sleep with your bedroom door closed, install an additional smoke detector in you room.

- Keep combustible materials away from your heating equipment, fireplaces, woodstoves etc.

- Chimneys should be inspected and cleaned if necessary once a year by a professional.

- If you install heating, cooking or electrical equipment be sure to get the proper permits and follow all installation codes.

- Store saturated cleaning rags in an air-tight container to avoid spontaneous combustion.

- When replacing a fuse, be sure the new fuse is the same amp size as the old.

- Portable and space heaters should be turned off when you leave a room. Also, keep heaters at least three feet from anything that can burn, including furniture, walls and people.

- Be careful when refueling a power mower. A hot mower and gasoline can be a deadly combination.

- Periodically check the cords and plugs on your appliances and lights. Replace cords that are frayed or cracked.

- Never run electrical cords under carpet.

- Always avoid overloading electrical outlets.

- Keep lighters and matches up high out of the reach of children, preferably in a locked cabinet.

- Wear short sleeves, or roll up long sleeves when cooking to avoid sleeve contact with a burner.

- Keep all pot and pan handles facing inward while cooking to avoid bumping them off the stove surface.

- Never leave cooking food unattended.

- When barbecuing, keep a water source nearby.

- When disposing of barbecue ashes, remember that even "cool" may be dangerous.

- Keep your stove and oven clean to avoid grease fires.

- Don't keep gasoline in your home. Store gasoline in an approved safety container outside in a shed or garage. Remember, gasoline fumes can travel throughout a room and be ignited by a pilot light or other open flame.

- Store all flammable liquids in labeled, metal containers and keep them away from heat and open flames.

- Don't use a flame or heat source inside a tent. Use a flashlight and be sure your tent is flame retardant.

- Make sure all escape paths (doors and windows) are easy to use.

Escape Plan

Plan to get out alive. Draw a floor plan of your home, including all doors and windows which may serve as exits **(see illustration 2)**. Determine two ways, a first and second choice, of escaping from each room. Your first choice should be the safest, fastest route, and the second choice should be used as an alternative in the event your first choice is blocked by fire or smoke. If you have second story bedrooms, your second way out may be through a window that leads to a porch or roof, or to an escape ladder that everyone knows how to use. Determine an outside meeting place like a tree, telephone pole or neighbor's home where all family members will meet after leaving your home during a fire. Then practice your escape plan with your entire family. **Practice at least twice a year.**

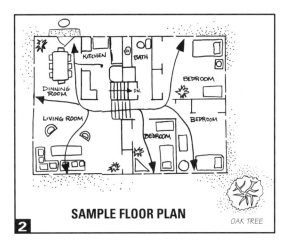

SAMPLE FLOOR PLAN

OAK TREE

2

During a Fire

Smoke Inhalation

In home fires, people are twice as likely to die of smoke inhalation as they are to die of burns. Smoke is your number one enemy in a fire.

The smoke, gasses and fumes released from burning materials in the average home are incredible. You can literally suffocate within minutes. The smoke is often thick, heavy and black, which means visibility, even in the light of day, may be next to nothing in a smoke filled home. Imagine yourself suddenly blind and unable to breathe in your home. What should you do?

Drop to the floor. Smoke rises, leaving a pocket of air at floor level. Your ability to breathe and see is greatly improved when you seek a crawling position in this smoke-free zone. The first rule then, if you encounter smoke while using your first escape route, is to turn around and use your second way out. If you must exit through smoke, DROP TO THE FLOOR AND CRAWL LOW UNDER THE SMOKE.

Feel Doors Before you Open Them

Feel closed doors before you open them. A hot or warm door may mean the next room is in flames, and open-ing the door could be disastrous. If a door is hot or warm, use your second way out. If escape is not possible, seal the cracks around the door with towels, tape or anything that will prevent smoke from entering. Then go to a window and signal for help. If there is a phone in the room, call the fire department and tell the dispatcher where you are.

If you leave a room, close the door behind you to help prevent the fire from spreading.

Get Out!

At the first sign of fire, shout **"Fire!"**, making sure everyone hears. Don't take time to get dressed or take time to gather possessions. Fire can spread extremely fast. Within seconds an entire room may be engulfed. That's why you shouldn't even take time to telephone for help. Get out. You can call the fire department from a neighbor's home once you're safely out of your home.

Stop, Drop and Roll

If you or your clothing catch fire, stop where you are, drop to the ground and roll over and over to extinguish the flames **(see illustration 3)**.

Summary

- At the first sign of a fire, alert your family by shouting **"Fire!"**

- If you are in a smoke-filled room, get down to the floor and crawl low under the smoke.

- Don't open doors that are hot or warm to the touch. Close all doors behind you.

- Get out of your home as quickly as possible. Don't get dressed. Don't gather

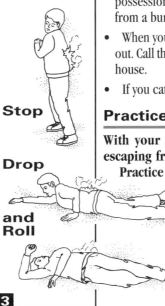

Stop

Drop

and Roll

3

possessions. Don't call the fire department from a burning building.

- When you are out of a burning building, stay out. Call the fire department from a neighbor's house.

- If you catch fire, **stop, drop and roll.**

Practice

With your family, practice all aspects of escaping from a fire at least twice a year. Practice crawling with your eyes closed to simulate the darkness you'll encounter during a real fire.

Hurricanes

Every year between the months of June and November hurricanes form in the North Pacific Ocean, the southern North Atlantic Ocean, the Caribbean Sea and the Gulf of Mexico. Because of geographic and weather factors, more hurricanes form in this area than anywhere in the world.

Hurricane history is rich with examples of destruction. Billions of dollars in property damage and thousands of lives have been claimed by hurricanes over the years. The most recent example of the incredible power of hurricanes was Hurricane Andrew. Striking both South Florida and the Gulf Coast of Louisiana on August 24th through the 26th, 1992, Hurricane Andrew proved to be the most damaging hurricane in U.S. history.

With winds from 135 to 165 miles per hour and a tidal surge of 8 feet, Hurricane Andrew ripped through South Florida taking 13 lives, leaving 250,000 people homeless and causing possibly as much as $20 billion in damage. Hurricane Andrew then plowed on through the Gulf of Mexico, slamming into the Louisiana coast with winds of 140 miles per hour, taking one life and causing extensive damage.

There's no question that hurricanes can cause extraordinary damage. But there are certain precautions you can take to protect yourself, and in many cases your home and belongings, from becoming a hurricane statistic.

Watches and Warnings

Despite our advanced technology, it's virtually impossible to predict precisely where a hurricane will strike land. It's possible though, to monitor a hurricane's development and estimate a coastal zone that it may strike.

A hurricane watch means that a hurricane is being monitored and there is the possibility that it could make landfall in 36 hours. Since it's a possibility, it's best to stay tuned to local hurricane information and be prepared to take further action.

A hurricane warning means that a hurricane is expected to make landfall within 24 hours. Stay tuned to local emergency information for further instructions.

Remember, you don't have to be directly in the path of a hurricane to be in danger. High surf and storm surge, gale force winds and heavy rains stretch out hundreds of miles from the eye of a hurricane.

Before a Hurricane

- Make sure you've assembled your survival supplies **(see Survival Supplies page 7)**. Emergency assistance may not be immediately available in the aftermath of a disaster. A three to seven day supply of food and water for each member of your family, as well as the other recommended supplies will make all the difference in the days following a hurricane.

- Keep your property free of debris. Lawn furniture, barbecue grills, tools and other items that aren't secured will most certainly be dangerous if they become airborne by winds exceeding 100 miles per hour. Tie down all items likely to become airborne. If you have time, shutter glass windows and doors with heavy plywood.

- Become familiar with the location of your local emergency shelter.

During a Hurricane

- Evacuate if told to do so. Take your emergency supplies with you. Over 2 million people had evacuated coastal areas of Florida and Louisiana in the hours before Hurricane Andrew. At the first word of a hurricane watch or warning, stay tuned to local emergency information for possible evacuation instructions.

- If you're unable to evacuate and your home has a basement, seek shelter there if you are sure it will not flood. Be sure to have survival supplies with you, and stay tuned to local hurricane information.

- If you're unable to evacuate and you don't have a basement, seek shelter away from windows, preferably under a heavy, sturdy table, or in an interior hallway or closet.

- Don't drive anywhere and don't go outside unless you're informed that the storm has passed. Remember, the eye of a hurricane is quiet.

- Don't misinterpret the eye of the hurricane for the end of the storm. If the eye passes over you, the hurricane will resume with just as much force as it previously had, sometimes even more.

After a Hurricane

- Continue to listen to hurricane emergency information and don't leave your shelter until you're told to do so. And then do so cautiously.

- When you return home check for structural damage like broken electrical lines or fixtures, and broken water and sewer lines. Also check your food supply for contamination.

- Administer first aid where needed.

- Help others, if you can (teamwork will be needed to clear debris).

- Don't drive anywhere unless absolutely necessary. Roads may be obstructed and dangerous and should be kept clear for emergency vehicles. Also, gasoline should be conserved.

- Don't use your telephone unless absolutely necessary.

Snow and Ice Storms

When people think of severe weather they think of tornados and hurricanes. That's because the damage they cause can be extremely visible. And yes, tornados and hurricanes take lives, but just as deadly (and in some cases even more deadly) are the quiet killers – snow, ice and cold.

Snow and ice storms are less sensational than more visible weather disasters, but each year snow and ice storms, along with cold temperatures, take hundreds of lives. The key to avoid becoming a statistic is simple – be prepared.

During the winter months, snow storms commonly occur throughout the United States. And although they're more common in the mid to upper latitude states, as well as higher altitudes, snow, ice and cold weather have been experienced by just about every community in the country at one time or another. That's

why everyone should at least know the basics of snow and ice storm preparedness no matter where you live.

Because this chapter deals with extreme cold temperatures, it's important that you use this chapter in conjunction with the chapter on Cold Exposure in the Priority One First Aid section **(page 103).**

Watches and Warnings

The National Weather Service issues watches and warnings to alert communities of potentially dangerous weather.

A winter storm watch means that conditions are right for certain severe weather conditions to occur. Stay tuned to local weather information for updates on changing conditions. Also, if possible, avoid traveling.

A winter storm warning means that severe weather exists and may be moving toward your area. Stay indoors. Travel only if it's absolutely necessary. Stay tuned to local weather information for updates on changing conditions.

Keep Warm

The reason for avoiding travel and staying indoors is that you'll reduce your risk of exposure to cold temperatures. However, if the heat in your house is not working and it's cold outside, leave your house and go to someplace warm. In the event of emergencies, your local Red Cross chapter may be able to refer you to a warming center. Also, you may want to have an emergency generator in your home to power your furnace, electrical appliances and lights. But consult your local gas or electric company first.

Survival Supplies

There is virtually no reason for you to leave the warmth of your home if you've assembled your survival supplies **(see Survival Supplies page 7)**. These survival supplies are meant to see you through emergencies like severe weather. If you haven't already studied this information and assembled your supplies, you should do so soon, or you may find yourself wishing you had.

Protect your Pipes

During times of extreme cold, exposed water pipes should be wrapped with insulation material, or even towels or rags to prevent freezing. Also, allowing faucets to drip keeps water flowing through pipes which helps prevent freezing.

Snow Shoveling

Many people take pride in keeping their sidewalks and driveways clear of snow and ice during the winter weather months. However, year after year, hundreds of people die from heart attacks while shoveling snow. Since shoveling snow is very strenuous, it's important to take many rest breaks. If you're elderly or have a heart condition, get help with your snow shoveling, especially with deep, heavy snow. Also, to avoid frostbite and hypothermia, wait until weather conditions have improved before shoveling snow. And always dress warmly.

Help your Neighbors

If you have elderly neighbors, check on them to make sure they're all right. If you're able, offer to shovel their snow. Again, sometimes pride gets in the way of asking for help. So offer your help.

The Dangers of Ice

Slippery sidewalks are simply a hazard. If you must walk anywhere, do so with caution.

Look Out for Power Lines

Ice storms have a tendency to bring down power lines. And because your body, as well as metal, and just about any moist or wet object is a good conductor of electricity, coming in contact with downed power lines can cause serious injury or even death. For this reason it's best to look out for and stay away from downed power lines.

If live power lines come in contact with your car and you're in it, stay inside your car until professional rescuers arrive. Most cars are insulated, providing protection from electricity as long as you avoid contact with metal parts of the car. Similarly, avoid rescuing anyone from a car that has come in contact with downed power lines.

Traveling

Never travel during serious winter weather unless it's absolutely necessary. If you must travel, always keep your gas tank full. Be sure your car is winterized with the proper anti-freeze. Keep survival supplies in your trunk **(see Automobile Survival Supplies page 13)** and always let someone know your destination and the exact route you will be taking, just in case you become stranded and they need to send help.

If you do become stranded, stay with your car. Start your car and let it run with the heater on for approximately 10 minutes per hour. Be sure your exhaust pipe is clear of snow. When your car is running, leave the dome light on so it's easier for your car to be seen. Keep a window that's not exposed to strong winds, open just a crack. Also, move your arms and legs frequently to keep blood circulating, which will help keep you warmer.

Tornadoes strike most often in the midwestern United States but can strike from the Rockies to the eastern seaboard. But no state is immune – tornadoes have touched down in every state in North America. And the force is deadly. Tornadoes occur most frequently during the months from March to June.

In April of 1965, 40 separate tornadoes struck the midwestern United States killing more than 270 people and causing over $190 million in property damage. The tornado that struck Wichita Falls, Texas in April of 1979 killed more than 60 people and caused over $400 million in property damage. And the list goes on, because year after year tornadoes take more lives and damage more property than any other weather related disaster.

A tornado is a severe low pressure storm which develops and strikes most often in the late afternoons and early evenings of warm, humid days in the spring and summer. It used to be that surviving a tornado depend- ed on chance, where you were when it struck. And today, chance is still an element when identifying where a tornado develops and touches down, but there's usually more warning time which means there's a greater chance for you to seek safety – and survive.

Tornado Watches and Warnings

The National Weather Service issues watches and warnings to alert communities of potentially dangerous weather.

A tornado watch means that conditions are right for a tornado to develop. Stay tuned to local weather information for updates on changing weather conditions. Also, if possible, avoid traveling.

A **tornado warning** means that a tornado has been sighted and may be moving toward your area. Stay indoors and seek shelter. Don't travel unless absolutely necessary. Stay tuned to local weather information for updates on changing weather conditions.

Shelter in your Home

If you're in your home or in a commercial building at the time of a tornado warning, the safest place for you to be is in the southwest corner of the basement. The southwest corner is optimum since tornadoes tend to move in that direction, taking debris with them, away from the southwest corner. For extra protection, you may want to get underneath a sturdy, heavy table or other covering. Stay there until you no longer hear the storm or the warning siren. Don't go upstairs to peek at the storm. Many people have died from curiosity.

If there's not a basement in the building that you're in, seek shelter underneath a table, desk or even a bed. Stay as close to the floor as possible. And stay away from windows which may shatter from airborne debris. In addition, take shelter in an interior hallway or closet away from windows and exterior doors.

TORNADOES

Shelter Outside

The winds of a tornado may blow in excess of 200 miles per hour, and the tornado itself may move at 30 to 50 miles per hour. If you are in an automobile when a tornado is approaching, get out of your automobile and lay flat in a ditch or low lying area. If there's no low lying area nearby, lay flat in an open area. Don't stand up. If you're on a highway or interstate, take cover under an overpass, up where the overpass and ground come together **(see illustration 4)**.

Survival Supplies

You should have already assembled your survival supplies in both your home and your automobile. Use your battery powered radio to keep informed of the tornado's development and to know when it's safe for you to leave your shelter. For a list of survival supplies as well as where to store them, **see Survival Supplies on page 7**.

If you have not already studied the Survival Supplies section or have not assembled your supplies, you should do so soon, or you may find yourself wishing you had.

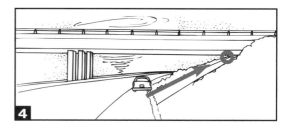

Burglary

In the United States alone, there are as many as 3 million household burglaries each year. And if you talk to anyone who has experienced a burglary of their home or apartment, they'll tell you it can be just as devastating, both mentally and monetarily, as most natural disasters.

Most people believe they and their belongings are safe within their home. A burglary, even an attempted break-in, can shatter that belief. And although some neighborhoods and some cities are statistically safer than others, today virtually every home and apartment in every city is at risk of burglary.

This chapter is designed to help you think the way a burglar thinks. By applying this thought process to your own house or apartment, you'll be able to discover weak spots – areas that make breaking in easier – and you'll be able to strengthen these weak spots which will not only discourage burglars, but will make you feel safer, more secure and less frightened.

Weak Spots

Burglars like to break in where it's easy to enter, easy to exit, and where they won't be seen. Areas particularly attractive to burglars include:

- Basement and ground floor entrances.

- Lightweight doors or single paned windows.

- Dark or poorly lit areas along the side of a house or in the back of a house, away from street and porch lights.

- Areas around a home that are secluded. Borders of trees, shrubs or a fence wall all provide needed cover for a burglar.

Lights, Locks and Alarms

By strengthening weak spots, you simply make your home or apartment less attractive to burglars. Keeping the area around your home well lit and as free from cover as possible, as well as strengthening doors and windows, will make a burglar's job more difficult, which will most likely disqualify your home or apartment in the burglar's mind.

Lights

A burglar wants to be invisible. Be sure all entrances are properly lit and that any front or side entrances are visible from the street. This includes illuminating sides of the house that are dark, and any back entrances. Lights may be simply switched on at dusk and off at dawn. However, some people prefer light sensitive outdoor lighting that automatically turns on at dusk and off at the first light of day, or motion sensitive lighting that automatically turns on when someone is approaching. The type of lighting you choose is based on personal preference. The important thing is that potential points of entry are illuminated.

Locks

If a burglar is bold enough to approach a well lit house, or is clever enough to find the one area least illuminated, your second line of defense includes strong locks. Examine every possible point of entry including all doors and windows – even old coal shoots and delivery doors. Be sure they're locked securely. Start with the basement and ground floor first, since this is the most vulnerable area, but don't ignore upper floors since they're not necessarily beyond a burglar's reach.

When selecting locks, dead bolt locks tend to be strongest, but a variety of door and window locks are available to suit your specific needs, and they're relatively easy to install. If you're not sure, check with your local police department for advice about good locks.

Alarms

Residential alarms are growing in popularity. Just the sight of a window sticker that displays the name of the alarm company is a deterrent to a burglar. Alarms range from extensive and elaborate protection covering all entries and internal motion detectors to simple door alarms. Most communities have at least one commercial alarm company that can answer specific questions on types of alarms and their effectiveness.

When you Leave Home for a Short Time

When you leave home for a short time, you need to take precautions. A burglar only needs a few minutes to get in and out of your house. And burglars that are more daring may even strike during daylight hours when neighbors may be less suspicious of their presence.

Keep the following things in mind before you leave:

- Lock all doors and windows, including garage doors.

- Keep lights on in the house and be sure the exterior of the house is well lit.

- Keep your curtains or blinds drawn at night so a burglar can't tell whether you're home or away. Also, keeping your curtains drawn prevents a burglar from seeing the contents of your house, which reduces temptation.

- Don't hide your keys anywhere outside your house. Have a friend or neighbor that you trust keep a spare set of keys for you.

- Bring inside any mail or newspapers that may have been delivered. These items left outside are a sign to burglars that you're not home.

- Never leave an announcement on your answering machine that lets callers know that you're out and when you'll be returning. A burglar may call to see if you're home. Leave a non-specific message like – "I'm busy and can't get to the telephone right now."

When you Leave Home for Vacation

Burglars look for easy targets and prefer to break in when no one is home. You can help "disqualify" your home from a burglar's mind by making it appear that you're home when you're actually away on vacation.

The most ideal situation is to hire a reputable house sitter, or have a friend stay at your house while you're away. Be sure to leave them with specific instructions on routine household care, as well as numbers where you can be reached. **If it's not possible for you to have a house sitter, keep the following things in mind:**

- Use timers to turn indoor lights on and off.

- Let friends and neighbors know that you'll be away. Ask them to "keep an eye" on your house while you're gone.

- Arrange for a friend or neighbor to bring your mail and any newspapers into the house on a daily basis. These items left outside are a sign to burglars that you're not home. Also, if possible, have them turn on different lights in your house and ask them to spend some time in your house, even a half hour an evening.

- Have a neighbor park in your driveway from time to time.

- Cut your lawn before you leave, and if you'll be away for more than a week, have a neighbor cut it when it gets long enough. An overgrown lawn suggests to a burglar that you're away.

- Never leave an announcement on your answering machine that lets callers know that you're out and when you'll be returning. A burglar may call to see if you're home. Leave a non-specific message like – "I'm busy and can't get to the telephone right now."

Documentation

Document your possessions for insurance purposes and for police investigators. Mark your valuables with your social security number, name and address. **Be sure to fill out the Property Profile forms at the back of this book.** Photograph and/or video tape your valuables, too. This will make it easier for police to identify them.

Coming Home to a Burglar

If you come home and notice that your home has been forcibly entered – don't go in. And if you don't realize your home has been broken into until you've entered – get out. Quickly go to a neighbor's house and call the police. Never sneak up on or surprise a burglar, no matter how angry you are. You never know if a burglar is armed or dangerous. Trying to stop a burglary could put an end to your life.

If you Hear a Burglar during the Night

Don't try to stop a burglar you hear at night in your house. If you're near a telephone, call the police. Locate something, preferably a blunt or heavy object, in order to protect yourself if necessary. Make noise, pretend to hold a conversation (even if you're alone). This will make the intruder believe there are more people in the house. But don't make your presence known if you have somehow blocked the intruder's exit.

Start a Neighborhood
Crime Watch Group

Organize neighbors to be on the lookout for anyone suspicious. These types of groups have been very effective in preventing burglary. For more information on organizing a group in your neighborhood, contact your local police department.

Personal Safety: Adults

Women, the elderly and young children are more vulnerable to personal attack than other groups. But realistically, no matter your size, build, race, age or sex, you are a potential victim of a personal attack. Most personal attacks take place in the evening hours, after sunset and before sunrise. Most attacks take place where there are few or no other people around, and in dark or poorly lit areas.

If you must travel alone, there are a number of things you can do to help prevent being attacked. But unfortunately, no matter how cautious you are, you may have to resort to self-defense techniques. This section covers both preventive measures you can take as well as the basics in self-defense.

Prevention

The best defense to surviving an attack is to avoid being targeted in the first place. There are many things you can do to help reduce your chances of being vulnerable.

Your Front Door

Personal attacks are known to be carried out by persons posing as workmen, deliverymen, people in need of help and acquaintances. So you need to be wary of anyone at your door.

- Be sure the area around your door is well lit so that people at your door can be seen by you and passers-by.

- If possible, look to see who's at your door, either through a window or through a peephole.

- If you can't see the person or can't identify them by their appearance, go to the door and ask who they are. Consider having a family or household policy of not opening the door to anyone you're not expecting.

- Install a peephole in your door. This will allow you to see who the person is and learn what they want. It's always best to be over cautious than not cautious enough.

- Don't put your full name on your mailbox or door bell. Use your last name and only your first initial if necessary. Attackers are more likely to attack a female living alone.

Keys and Locks

Don't hide your keys anywhere outside your house. Have a friend or neighbor that you trust keep a spare set of keys for you. When inside your house, be sure to lock all doors behind you.

Your Telephone

A potential attacker may use your telephone as a means to discover who you are, and to learn if you're at home.

Never give your telephone number to a stranger that calls. If you're having problems with strangers calling, you may want to consider using an answering machine to "screen" your calls, having your telephone number unlisted or changed, calling the police, or checking with your local telephone company to see what other services are available to help you.

Out and About

Most attackers strike people walking alone at night in dark or poorly lit places. There are a number of common sense precautions you can take based on this information alone. But the general rule is to be aware of your surroundings.

- Try to walk with others. If you're in a situation where you don't have anyone else to walk with, choose a busy route – a route that ensures other people will always be in sight.

- Walk in well lit areas. Don't take short-cuts through alleys, dark parks or areas that are unfamiliar to you.

- Keep your distance from people who seem menacing or suspicious, but avoid reacting to stereotypes. Act on your "gut" feelings. Cross the street if you have to.

- Always carry change for public telephones as well as the telephone numbers of friends and taxi companies. You can call 9-1-1 free from most pay phones.

- Keep alert. Always keep a watchful eye for suspicious looking people and always be aware of your surroundings. Being alert and confident, and showing it as you walk, is a deterrent to attackers.

Automatic Teller Machines

Be aware of the area surrounding your ATM. If something is suspicious, use a different ATM. Take a friend with you if you use an ATM at night, and be sure to park in a well-lit area. Put your cash away immediately.

Automobile

Even though you're safer from attack while driving alone in your car than while walking alone at night, "car-jacking" and attacks on motorists have been steadily rising in recent years. Again, being aware of your surroundings is your first rule of defense.

- Plan your route. Let family and friends know the route you're taking. Let them know when you're leaving and when you expect to return.

- Before you leave, make sure your car is in good working order and make sure you have a full tank of gas. Carry a survival kit in your trunk at all times. **(see Automobile Survival Supplies page 13).**

- Keep your doors locked and windows rolled up while you're in your car.

- Don't stop and get out of your car in areas that you don't feel safe. Always be aware of your surroundings before you unlock your door and get out of your car.

- Don't give rides to strangers.

- Identify businesses along your most frequently traveled routes at which you could stop if you needed help.

Self-defense

No matter how cautious you may be, you're still vulnerable to attack. Many attackers are robbers or "muggers". If you're confronted by a stranger who demands money, jewelry or valuables – don't resist. Simply hand over what they want. No valuables are worth more than your life.

Many attackers perpetrate violence such as rape and racial attacks. Again, the best way to prepare for these types of situations is to reduce your vulnerability. But since this isn't always possible to do, self-defense maneuvers may be necessary.

Self-defense techniques are best learned by taking a credible self-defense class. Your local police department is a good place to begin learning about the classes offered in your area. There are a number of basic self-defense maneuvers you can use, however, if classes are not offered in your area.

Weapons

If it's legal where you live, you may want to consider carrying a chemical spray. This can temporarily blind attackers or cause difficulty breathing, providing you with a chance to escape. Also, compact, compressed-air alarms are sold commercially which sound an incredibly loud noise. If confronted by a potential attacker, these types of alarms may not only deafen and startle the attacker, they may alert others that something is wrong. The problem with weapons is that many are not legal to carry, you may not have enough time to use them especially if the attack is a complete surprise, they may mechanically fail, and any weapon may be taken by the attacker and used against you.

Physical Force

In many cases, basic self-defense maneuvers may be your only weapon when under attack. The objective of self-defense maneuvers is to temporarily disable your attacker so you can get away before you're harmed.

- **Look angry** — let your attacker immediately know that you're angry and that you won't tolerate any abuse. In many cases, by giving your attacker your angriest look, you will have an immediate psychological advantage.

- **Sound angry** — loud yells of anger are not only unexpected and disorienting to your attacker, but they also help to attract the attention of everyone else in the area.

- **Strike decisively** — the human body has a number of weak or vulnerable points. They include the eyes, nose, throat, kidneys, knee caps and in male attackers – the groin. Quickly select and strike one point (or as many as you can) in order to disable your attacker **(see illustration 5)**. It's important that you don't just hurt your attacker, which may make him angrier and more violent. Strike quickly and strike decisively as many times as possible. Then escape from the scene as quickly as you can.

5

Personal Safety: Children

It's unfortunate but true that today the abduction and exploitation of children is a regular occurrence. That's why it's important to teach your children about abduction. If you teach them while they're young as you teach them other coping skills, they'll view prevention as natural and will less likely be frightened by the idea.

Communicate with your Children

Children are uniquely vulnerable. Since it's impossible to be with your child all day to protect them, it's important to create an atmosphere in your home that makes it easy for your children to talk to you about what's going on in their lives. If your child feels comfortable talking to you about a sensitive matter, you'll be able to detect problems and protect your child before a situation worsens.

Be Prepared

- Be sure to have current photographs of your child on hand. A child under seven should be photographed at least every six months. A child over seven should be photographed at least every year.

- If possible, videotape your child.

- Maintain up-to-date dental records of your child.

- If possible, have your child's fingerprints taken.

- Fill out Personal Profile forms at the back of this book.

Be Aware

- Always know the whereabouts of your child and who they're with.

- Be aware and suspicious of any "grown-up" that's spending too much time and attention on your child.

- Don't write your child's name on their things (lunch boxes, clothes etc.). This will help prevent a stranger from knowing your child's name.

- Know the exact route your child takes to and from school.

- Get involved. Know who your child's friends are, where they go and what they do.

- Be careful about choosing a babysitter or daycare service. Ask for references and check them.

- Never leave your child alone in your car.

- Listen to your child's fears. If they don't want to spend time with someone, find out why. Communicate.

Teach your Child

- Teach your child what are appropriate and inappropriate requests from adults.

- Teach your child never to go anywhere with anyone, unless you've given them permission.

- If they become separated from you, teach them to ask someone who works where they are lost to help find you. They shouldn't wander around alone looking for you.

- Teach your child to not go anywhere alone.

- Teach your child to memorize their full name, address, telephone number, your work telephone number and area code. Practice with your child periodically.

- An adult should never ask your child to keep a secret. Your child should tell you if this occurs.

- A child should say **"no"** to anyone who makes them feel uncomfortable, and they should shout for help if they're being threatened.

- Teach your child that they should never open a door to strangers.

- If they are being followed, a child should not hide. They should go to a place where people are, like to a store or a neighbor's house, and ask for help.

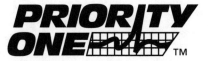

First Aid

Introduction

The Priority One First Aid Guide may someday play a role in saving a life. If you consider that 9 out of 10 people will visit an emergency department in their lifetime, either escorting a family member or friend, or for their own medical emergency, there's a good chance that you'll someday need the Priority One First Aid Guide. This guide is helpful even for minor emergencies like a sprained ankle or cut finger.

First aid is the help you give prior to seeking professional medical attention. The Priority One First Aid Guide is meant to provide basic information about the most commonly occurring injuries so that you may provide assistance in a timely manner.

This guide is not necessarily meant to be read from cover to cover. However, the first several sections should be read now in order to prepare you for first aid situations.

Also, The Priority One First Aid Guide is not meant to replace any formal course in first aid. In fact, we urge you to take courses that can better prepare you for emergency medical situations. Your local Red Cross chapter or American Heart Association affiliate is a good place to seek information about the courses that are available in your community.

The following "guidelines" should be used in conjunction with specific recommendations from your personal physician.

Before an Emergency

Buy a First Aid Kit

There are a large variety of commercial first aid kits available. Most contain only the supplies needed for the most commonly occurring first aid procedures. Be sure to have a first aid kit in your home and car and get to know the contents of your first aid kit, so when the time comes to use it for a real emergency you won't waste any time choosing the proper items.

Your First Aid Kit Should at Least Contain:

First Aid Supplies

- ☐ Sterile adhesive bandages in assorted sizes
- ☐ Hypoallergenic adhesive tape (1-2 rolls)
- ☐ 8 inch x 10 inch combination dressings (4)
- ☐ 2 inch sterile gauze pads (4-6)
- ☐ 4 inch sterile gauze pads (4-6)
- ☐ 2 inch sterile roller bandages (3 rolls)
- ☐ 3 inch sterile roller bandages (3 rolls)
- ☐ Triangular bandages (3)
- ☐ Antiseptic
- ☐ Cleansing agent/soap
- ☐ Pre-moistened towelettes (10)
- ☐ Tongue blades (2)
- ☐ Lightweight shock blanket (1)
- ☐ Watertight medication container (1)
- ☐ Thermometer (1)
- ☐ Tweezers (1)
- ☐ Scissors (1)

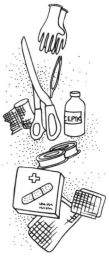

- [ ] Latex gloves (2 pair)
- [ ] Needle
- [ ] Assorted sizes of safety pins
- [ ] Tube of petroleum jelly or other lubricant (1)

Non-prescription Drugs for your First Aid Kit

(Be sure to check and rotate according to expiration dates)

- [ ] Aspirin or non-aspirin pain reliever
- [ ] Anti-diarrhea medication
- [ ] Antacid (for stomach upset)
- [ ] Syrup of Ipecac (use to induce vomiting if advised by the Poison Control Center)
- [ ] Laxative
- [ ] Activated charcoal (use if advised by the Poison Control Center)

Where to Keep your First Aid Kit

Keep your first aid kit out of the way but within easy reach. Your first aid kit should be neat and organized. Don't use it as an extension of your medicine cabinet, or as a storage place for unrelated items. For this reason, and to protect children, keep your first aid kit out of the way of your daily life. But don't hide it away. You should always know exactly where it is. And it should be in easy reach when you need it. The time you save in locating your first aid kit is time that may make a big difference in someone's health.

Know your Numbers

You and your first aid kit alone can't take care of all emergencies. In fact, a big part of first aid is seeking the proper medical attention. More often than not, part of your first aid giving includes picking up a telephone and calling for further assistance. Whether it be your doctor or your local emergency medical service (EMS), you must always be prepared to pick up a telephone and dial quickly.

Make a list of important numbers and keep it near your telephone. The list should include your own address and telephone number in case someone not familiar with them (like a baby sitter or neighbor) is making the call.

At the back of this guide there is a list of important telephone numbers and personal medical profile forms. Be sure to complete this information soon, before an emergency happens.

EMS

This symbol (EMS) appears throughout The Priority One First Aid Guide. It's meant to inform you that the situation may be very serious and you should call for EMS (emergency medical services). In most communities, EMS may be contacted by simply dialing 9-1-1 **(see 9-1-1 page 70).** If your community doesn't have the 9-1-1 system, contact the emergency medical services used by your community (police department, fire department or local ambulance service). **If you are ever in doubt of the severity of a medical condition, we strongly urge you to call EMS.**

Spinal Injury

If ever you suspect a spinal, neck or back injury, don't move the victim unless absolutely necessary. **(For more information see Spinal Injury page 83.)** Contact EMS immediately. Give first aid for life-threatening injuries only, (injuries which cause a person to not breathe or have a pulse) and then do so as gently as possible, so as not to disturb the victim's position.

Check for Medical Alert Tag

Many people have certain medical conditions that make them susceptible to illness. As a first aid giver, the more information you have about what's wrong with a victim, the easier it will be for you and medical professionals to help. As part of assessing a first aid situation, always remember to check the victim for a medical alert tag which may be worn around the wrist, neck, or ankle.

Moods are Contagious

Try to prepare yourself mentally for an emergency. An emergency medical situation can happen to anyone, at any time. It's very important that you remain calm while giving first aid. If you're scared or excited, you can easily spread your anxiety to the injured person, making them scared or excited. And that can actually make their condition worse. Be realistic, but be as reassuring as possible.

9-1-1

Many communities have a 9-1-1 system, the three digit telephone number that quickly connects you to police, fire and emergency medical services (EMS). Using 9-1-1 can save several minutes – a long time when an emergency is taking place. But remember, 9-1-1 should only be dialed for police, fire and medical service when emergency response is needed. Don't dial 9-1-1 for routine law enforcement, fire or medical questions.

When you dial 9-1-1, remember to remain calm and speak clearly. Be prepared to provide the 9-1-1 communications specialist with the following information:

- **What is happening**
- **The address, nearest cross-street(s), and your name**
- **The telephone number you're calling from**

Be prepared to stay on the telephone to give any other information needed.

Always be patient while the 9-1-1 communications specialist is asking you questions. Remember that he or she is a professional, and every question asked is necessary to ensure a safe, quick response to your emergency. In many cases, help has already been dispatched before the communications specialist begins to ask you for additional information.

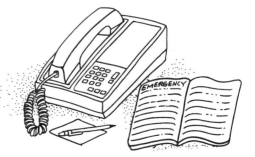

CPR

Cardiopulmonary resuscitation (CPR) can be life-saving, but it's best performed by people trained in a CPR course. We urge you to take a CPR course, which is offered by your local Red Cross chapter or American Heart Association affiliate. **The following information is not meant to replace a course in CPR – it's meant instead to inform you of the basics in the event you need to perform CPR between the time you read this information and the time you take an official course.**

Cardiopulmonary means "heart" and "lungs." Cardiopulmonary resuscitation combines rescue breathing to provide oxygen to the victim's lungs, where it can be taken up by the blood, with chest compressions to circulate the oxygen-carrying blood. Without oxygen, brain cells begin to die within four to six minutes.

EMS **If the victim isn't breathing or has no pulse, call 9-1-1 for help through the emergency medical services (EMS) system. If assistance is nearby, shout for someone else to call EMS. If the victim is under 8 years of age, you're trained in CPR, and there's no one available to call EMS, administer CPR for 1 minute and then call EMS yourself.**

EMS **If you have any doubt about your ability to administer CPR, call for EMS. The EMS or 9-1-1 communications specialist is often able to provide CPR instructions over the phone.**

1. With the help of people around you, position the victim on their back and on a firm surface (not a bed) so you can administer CPR. If you suspect spinal injury, slowly and gently roll the victim onto his or her back, keeping the victim's head, neck and back supported and aligned.

2. Check for responsiveness to verbal and non-verbal stimuli. Get down beside the victim's ear and ask loudly "Are you ok?" If they don't respond, shake the victim's shoulders firmly without moving the head or neck.

3. Check the victim's ABCs **(Airway, Breathing and Circulation)**.

Airway

Open the airway by placing one hand on the victim's forehead and two fingers of the other hand under the victim's chin. Gently tilt the victim's head back while lifting up on the chin **(see illustration 6).** If you suspect the victim has suffered a spinal injury, gently lift the chin without tilting the head back. If this doesn't open the airway, tilt the head back just a little.

Breathing

Put your ear close to the victim's mouth and listen and feel for signs of breathing **(see illustration 7).** If there are no signs of breathing, pinch the soft part of the victim's nose shut and close your lips over the victim's mouth **(see illustration 8).** Give two slow, full breaths. Observe the victim's chest to see that it rises with each breath. If the victim's chest doesn't rise between each breath, repeat the steps to open the airway. If the victim's chest still doesn't rise, look in the mouth for an obstruction.

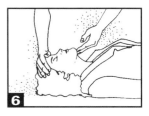

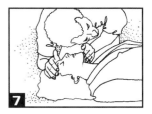

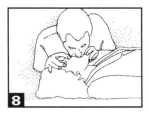

Circulation

Feel for the pulse from the carotid artery on the victim's neck **(see illustration 9).** Don't use your thumb to feel for a pulse. Take a moment now to feel your own pulse

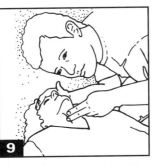

so that you will know where to locate it on the victim.

4. At this point, if the victim is breathing and you can feel a pulse, stay with the victim until EMS help arrives. Also, give first aid for other injuries and continue to monitor ABCs.

5. If the victim has a pulse but little or no breathing, continue giving breaths as before, until EMS help arrives. Be sure to monitor the victim's pulse **(see step 6 below).**

6. If the victim has no pulse, prepare to administer chest compressions by kneeling at the side of the victim's chest and centering the palm of your hand over the victim's breast bone, with the edge of your

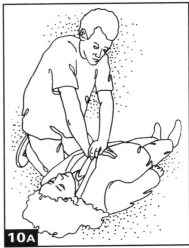

hand about one inch above the lower tip of the victim's breastbone **(see illustration 10A).** Cover the back of the hand on the chest with your free hand.

Be sure that your shoulders are directly over the victim's chest with your arms straight **(see illustration 10B).** Pivoting from your hips, push down on the breast bone, depress-

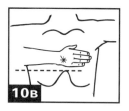

ing the chest approximately two inches (adults) with 15 smooth thrusts a little faster than one per second.

7. Reopen the airway by placing one hand on the victim's forehead and again lift the victim's chin. Give two slow full breaths (as described above).

8. Repeat steps 5 and 6 three more times

9. Recheck the ABCs. If the victim is breathing and you can feel a pulse, stay with the victim until EMS help arrives. Also, give first aid for other injuries and continue to monitor ABCs.

10. If you can feel a pulse but the victim isn't breathing, continue rescue breathing.

11. If you can't feel a pulse and the victim shows no signs of breathing after the first CPR cycle, continue giving CPR with 15 compressions and 2 breaths per cycle as in steps 5 and 6.

Again, the preceding information is not meant to replace a course in CPR. We urge you to take an official CPR course.

Bleeding

Loss of blood can be serious, so it's important to get bleeding under control as quickly as possible. Scrapes, cuts and other minor wounds will naturally clot and stop bleeding. Serious wounds, however, may bleed so rapidly that clots will not form. With serious wounds, direct pressure is the key to controlling blood loss.

Arteries carry blood away from the heart, while veins carry blood back to the heart. Arterial bleeding is life threatening since bright red blood will spurt from the wound with each beat of the heart. Bleeding from a vein can also be serious, but the flow is steady (not spurting) and a darker color. Severe bleeding may occur if a large artery or vein is involved, or if many smaller vessels are damaged (such as on the face or scalp). The amount of bleeding is not the only determinant of the seriousness of a laceration or cut – seriousness is also determined by the size (length and depth) and

damage to nerves, tendons and other structures around the wound.

Several infectious diseases can be spread by direct contact with blood to an open wound. It is therefore always advisable to use gloves when providing first aid for bleeding. Also, every attempt should be made to prevent blood from getting into your eyes or mouth.

External Bleeding, Lacerations and Cuts

EMS **If the wound is serious or bleeding is severe (even if you have it under control), call EMS.**

- **Don't probe a wound to see how deep it is.**

- **Don't remove anything embedded in a wound.**

- **Don't clean or disturb a wound after you have bleeding under control.**

1. Wash your hands and wear latex gloves if possible.

2. Remove any loose debris from the wound surface, but don't remove anything embedded in the wound.

3. If the wound is serious, apply direct pressure by placing a thick pad of clean, dry gauze (or any clean substitute – a towel, shirt, etc.) directly over the wound. If the wound is gaping, close it by pressing its edges together, then apply direct pressure. While applying pressure, try to keep the wound raised above the level of the victim's heart. If the gauze pad becomes soaked with blood, don't remove it from the wound - lay a fresh pad directly over the soaked one and keep applying pressure.

4. If bleeding doesn't stop after applying pressure for 15 minutes, and you are a long way from medical assistance, call for help and consider using pressure point bleeding control. For an arm wound, apply direct pressure to the artery between the two mus-cles on the inside of the arm until you no longer feel a pulse under your fingers **(see illustration 11A)**. For a leg wound, apply direct pressure to the artery at the crease between the top of the leg and the abdomen **(see illustration 11B)**.

5. Cover the victim with a blanket or anything handy that will keep the victim warm and help prevent shock **(see Shock page 81)**.

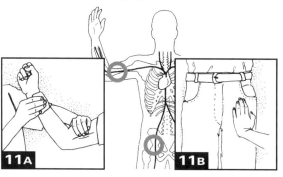

6. If the wound is minor, clean and bandage the wound **(see Cleaning and Bandaging Wounds page 78)**.

7. The sight of blood may frighten the victim. Try to keep the victim calm and relaxed.

Internal Bleeding

Internal bleeding can be life-threatening, but it is sometimes difficult to detect. Internal bleeding is often associated with broken bones, or when the body receives a hard blow.

Signs of internal bleeding include abdominal pain or swelling; blood in vomit, stool, urine, or coming from the vagina; bruises on the chest, abdomen, or hips, and/or weakness.

EMS **If you think the victim is suffering from internal bleeding, call EMS.**

• **Don't give the victim anything to eat or drink, including any medicine.**

1. Check the victims ABCs. If you need to, begin rescue breathing and/or CPR **(see CPR pages 71-74)**. Get medical help.

2. Cover the victim with a blanket or anything handy that will keep the victim warm and help prevent shock **(see Shock page 81)**.

3. If the victim vomits and you don't suspect a spinal injury, quickly turn the victim to his or her side.

4. Stay with the victim until medical help arrives.

Cleaning and Bandaging Wounds

It's important to clean and bandage a wound in order to prevent infection. Bandages also help to control bleeding and promote healing. The type of bandage you make depends on the size of the wound and where it's located. This section concentrates on the basic principles of cleaning and bandaging various types of wounds. When you become familiar with the basics, you'll be able to improvise in order to accommodate just about any wound you may encounter.

Cleaning a Wound

A minor wound should be cleaned to remove contamination before it is dressed and bandaged. Anything that you use to clean the wound and anything that comes in contact with the wound should be as clean as possible (preferably sterile).

EMS If a wound is deep and bleeding severely, don't clean it. Apply a pressure bandage to control bleeding (see Bleeding pages 75-76) and call EMS.

EMS If you can't clean a wound thoroughly, bandage it and get medical help.

1. Wash your hands and wear latex gloves if possible.

2. Clean the wound with soap and warm water.

3. Dry the wound by blotting it with sterile gauze. If the wound is minor and you feel medical help isn't necessary, apply a small amount of antibiotic ointment and then bandage the wound. It is important to assure that the victim's tetanus immunization status is up to date – he/she should check with their physician.

The Basic Bandage

A bandage actually has two parts: the dressing and the outer bandage. The dressing is a sterile covering placed over the wound; the bandage holds the dressing in place and supports the injured area. The "Band-Aid®", for example, is a dressing and bandage in one. "Band-Aids" are ideal for most small, minor cuts and scrapes. For larger wounds, you will have to create your own bandage with sterile dressings and tape from your first aid kit. However, if these items are not available, you may have to improvise with clean household linen or clean cloth for dressings, and cloth ties, adhesive tape, and even masking tape for the bandage.

1. After cleaning a wound, select or cut a sterile gauze dressing that's just a little larger than the wound.

2. Apply the dressing directly over the wound. Don't slide the dressing into place.

3. Secure the dressing in place with tape or with a bandage. Be sure the bandage fits securely but doesn't restrict circulation.

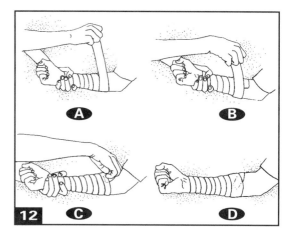

The Roller Bandage Technique

For wounds on an arm, leg, chest or abdomen, use a roller bandage instead of tape. A roller bandage is simply wrapped over the dressing and around the limb with spiral turns, starting at the narrowest part and moving up. Each turn should cover at least half of the last one. Tuck the end of the bandage under the last full turn and secure it with a safety pin or tape **(see illustration 12)**. Be sure the bandage fits securely but doesn't restrict circulation. You can test this by pressing your thumb firmly against the skin over a finger or toe below the bandage and then releasing the pressure. The skin should go from white to pink/red within a few seconds.

Shock

Shock happens when the body's flow of blood is reduced, resulting in too little oxygen flowing to the body's cells. Shock can be caused by many things, including severe bleeding, dehydration, hypothermia (low body temperature), heat illness, heart failure, burns, drug overdose and low blood sugar. It is easier to prevent shock than to treat it once it happens. That's why it's important to give first aid for the illness or injury that causes shock as soon as possible, so that the shock does not worsen.

Symptoms of shock include skin which is pale, moist, and cold (especially the arms, legs, and face), a fast heartbeat and rapid breathing, and dizziness or feeling faint when trying to sit or stand up.

The body expends energy and oxygen trying to keep warm – oxygen it doesn't have to spare when shock occurs. For this reason, it is important to keep the patient from losing additional body heat. Lying on a cold surface can cause heat loss up to 25 times faster than the cold air around the victim, so it is as critical to put a blanket or clothing underneath the victim as it is to cover them.

EMS **If the symptoms of shock are present or you're not sure call EMS.**

- **Don't give the victim anything to eat or drink.**

- **Don't raise the victim's head (i.e., with a pillow).**

1. Check the victims ABCs. If you need to, begin rescue breathing and/or CPR **(see CPR pages 71-74)**. Get medical help.

2. Try to determine the cause of shock. Check the victim for a medical alert tag.

3. Don't move the victim if you suspect head, neck, back, or spinal injury; or if the victim is having difficulty breathing. If you suspect spinal injury or are not sure, assume the victim has a spinal injury – Go to Step 5 below and **see Spinal Injury page 83**.

4. If you do not suspect spinal injury, place the victim in the shock position **(see illustration 13)**. Place a blanket or clothing on the ground, then lay the victim flat on their back and elevate their feet 8-12 inches. Use books, pillows, or anything handy to raise the victim's feet, but don't raise the victim's head. If this position makes the victim uncomfortable, or if they develop difficulty breathing, lower the legs to ground level.

5. Give first aid for any underlying illness or injury.

6. Loosen any restrictive clothing and cover the victim with a blanket or anything handy that will keep them warm.

7. If the victim is drooling or vomits and you do not suspect spinal injury, turn the victim's head to one side so that fluids can drain (if you suspect spinal injury, **see Spinal Injury page 83**).

8. Stay with the victim and continue to monitor ABCs until medical help arrives.

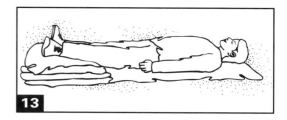

13

Spinal Injury

The spinal cord is made up of nerve tissue that runs through the center of the backbone. This nerve tissue is essential for controlling the entire body. You can injure your spine by injuring the muscles, ligaments, bones and nerves in your neck and back.

A serious injury to the neck or back can lead to paralysis. That's why it's important as a first aid giver to always be on the look out for possible neck or back injury. And if you ever suspect such an injury – even if you're not sure – it's important to keep the victim as still as possible to avoid making the injury worse. In other words, don't move a victim who may have a neck or back injury, unless absolutely necessary. Keep the victim still until medical help arrives.

Signs and symptoms of spinal injury include pain in the head, neck, back and/or abdomen; tingling or loss of feeling in an arm or leg; paralysis; and shock. The two most important first aid procedures when you suspect a spinal injury are to call EMS and to not move the victim.

EMS **Call EMS**

- **Don't move the victim in any way unless the victim is in a dangerous situation, they are not breathing, or they have no pulse.**

1. Keep the victim absolutely still.

2. Treat the victim for any obvious injuries.

3. Check the victim's ABCs **(see CPR pages 71-74).** Open the airway, check breathing and circulation. If necessary begin rescue breathing and/or CPR **(see CPR pages 71-74).** If the victim isn't laying on his or her back, you'll have to move the victim in order to begin CPR or rescue breathing. With the help of people around you, slowly and gently roll the victim as a unit onto his or her back, keeping the victim's head, neck and back supported and in-line.

4. If the victim's ABCs are present, keep the victim as still as possible. Support the victim's head and neck with your hands, with pillows, blankets or anything that will help keep the victim's head and neck in line and from moving.

5. If the victim is vomiting or choking on fluids, slowly and gently roll the victim onto his or her side, keeping the victim's head, neck and back supported and in-line. And again, if you have to move the victim, do so with the help of people around you.

6. Cover the victim with a blanket, or anything handy to keep the victim warm and to help prevent shock.

7. Wait with the victim, keeping him or her still, until help arrives.

Unconsciousness

A person may become unconscious from just about any serious injury or illness. There are many different levels of unconsciousness, ranging from drowsiness to total collapse. The first step is to assess the patient's state of responsiveness to verbal and non-verbal (shake and shout) stimuli. If they do not awaken readily, or if they slide back into unconsciousness, your two most important first aid procedures are to: (1) get medical help and (2) obtain and maintain an open airway until medical help arrives **(see Airway in CPR section page 72)**.

EMS The first aider must be aware of life-threatening hazards such as electrical wires or noxious gases prior to assessing the patient. If any life-threatening hazards exist, call EMS and wait for trained personnel to rescue the victim.

EMS Always call EMS for any person who is unconscious and cannot be awakened readily.

- **Don't leave an unconscious victim alone except to call EMS.**

- **Don't give the victim anything by mouth, even after they revive, before first consulting a physician.**

1. Check for responsiveness to verbal and non-verbal stimuli. Get down beside the victim's ear and ask loudly "Are you ok?" If they don't respond, shake the victim's shoulders firmly without moving the head or neck.

2. Check the victims ABCs. If you need to, begin rescue breathing and/or CPR **(see CPR pages 71-74)**. Get medical help.

3. If the victim's ABCs are present and you don't suspect a spinal injury, place the victim in the recovery position – on their side, with the face turned down to allow secretions to drain **(see illustration 14)**.

4. If the victim's ABCs are present and you do suspect a spinal injury, leave the victim in the position they were found until medical help arrives. You may need to lift the chin firmly **(see Airway page 72)** to maintain the airway.

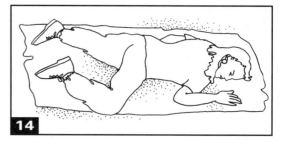

14

5. Look for evidence of underlying medical illnesses such as medications or a Medic Alert Tag.

6. Unless the victim feels hot, cover them with a blanket or anything handy that will keep them warm and help prevent shock.

7. Gently restrain the victim if the victim becomes restless. If the victim has seizures, give first aid for seizures **(see Seizures page 123)**.

Allergic Reaction

An allergic reaction can happen to just about anyone at just about any time. It can be caused by something swallowed (like seafood, nuts, or some drugs), something in the air (like pollen), or it can develop after being bitten or stung by an insect. If you suspect that the allergic reaction was caused by an insect, **see Bites and Stings page 89.**

Allergic reaction symptoms include itching, hives, a flushed or red face (or skin), dizziness and weakness, swelling of the eyes, face or tongue, nausea and vomiting, abdominal pain, wheezing, and difficulty breathing.

Mild allergic reactions often appear with just hives and itching. Typically in these cases, the body will win its fight with the offending substance, and no emergency care or medications will be needed as long as the victim has no further contact with the thing or substance that caused the reaction. Be sure to watch the victim closely for any signs of the condition worsening (i.e., problems breathing, throat tightness, unconsciousness).

Severe (anaphylactic) reactions are characterized by throat tightness, breathing difficulties, generalized swelling or unconsciousness. In the presence of a severe allergic reaction, EMS should be called immediately. If possible, the victim should be removed from further contact with the allergen and the ABCs should be assessed. Shock and unconsciousness should be treated as outlined **(see Shock page 81 and Unconsciousness page 85).** Allergic individuals may carry an anaphylaxis kit that contains emergency medications – in severe reactions, the self-injection of adrenaline (epinephrine) can be life-saving.

EMS **If the allergic reaction is severe, or a mild reaction is getting worse (problems breathing, throat tightness, unconsciousness), call EMS.**

- **Don't give the victim anything by mouth unless told to do so by a medical professional.**

1. Check the victims ABCs. If you need to, begin rescue breathing and/or CPR **(see CPR pages 71-74)**. Get medical help.

2. Try to keep the victim calm and relaxed.

3. Determine what it was that caused the reaction and be sure the victim has no further contact with it.

4. If the patient is having a severe reaction and they have an anaphylaxis kit prescribed by their doctor, help them give themselves the injection of adrenaline (epinephrine).

5. Cover the victim with a blanket or anything handy that will keep the victim warm and help prevent shock. If necessary, give further first aid to prevent shock **(see Shock page 81)**.

6. If the victim loses consciousness, give first aid for unconsciousness **(see Unconsciousness page 85)**.

7. Stay with the victim until medical help arrives.

8. Treat for shock if signs are present **(see Shock page 81)**.

Bites and Stings

Most insect bites and stings are minor and don't require professional medical attention. All insect bites and stings should be treated to prevent infection, and should be monitored since some people may develop an allergic reaction **(see Allergic Reaction page 87)** or disease. If it's possible, without causing harm to you or the victim, try to identify the insect. Bite and sting signs and symptoms range from clearly visible holes or stinger in the skin to itching, swelling and redness.

Animal bites are more serious. These wounds should be treated for bleeding, bandaged, and medical attention should be sought promptly.

EMS **If the victim is having difficulty breathing, is wheezing, faints, develops abdominal pain, or has been stung in the mouth or throat, call EMS.**

EMS **If the victim is rapidly developing an allergic reaction, call EMS, and then refer to the Allergic Reaction section (see page 87).**

Stings

Bee, Hornet, and Wasp Stings

Bee, hornet and wasp stings are common summertime injuries. Reactions can be mild or severe. Mild reactions consist of local swelling and itching and may be treated with a cold compress. More severe reactions include hives and severe allergic reactions. The latter can be life-threatening and may require the administration of adrenaline (epinephrine) if the patient has a bee-sting (anaphylaxis) kit prescribed by a physician. Honey bees leave a stinger in the skin and this must be removed as early as possible to prevent continued exposure to bee venom. Don't remove a honey bee stinger with a tweezers or by pinching it – squeezing the stinger may inject more venom into the victim.

1. Check the victims ABCs. If you need to, begin rescue breathing and/or CPR **(see CPR pages 71-74)**. Get medical help.

2. Watch for signs of shock and treat for shock if necessary **(see Shock page 81)**.

3. Keep the victim calm.

4. If a stinger is seen in the skin it should be removed as early as possible by scraping it off with a blunt edge like a recipe card or credit card.

5. Clean the wound with soap and water. Use a disinfectant if available.

6. To reduce pain and swelling, apply a cold compress (a towel soaked in cold water or wrapped around a bag of ice) to the wound area.

7. Keep the area around the wound free of any tight clothing and remove jewelry since swelling may occur.

8. Monitor the victim for signs that the condition may be worsening such as problems breathing or swelling of the mouth or face.

Tick Bites

Ticks burrow slowly under the skin and may only be visible as a small dark spot.

Do not forcefully remove a tick from under the skin since you can't be sure you've removed all of it. Get medical help.

1. If the tick remains on the surface of the skin, remove it with a tweezers, grasping the tick firmly and close to the skin, but don't crush or squeeze it. Pull the tick out with a steady, easy motion. Be sure to remove all of the tick, including the head and mouth parts. You may need to use a magnifying glass.

2. If you can't remove all of the tick, get medical help.

3. Clean the wound with soap and water. Use a disinfectant if available.

4. Monitor the victim for any signs of infection or disease. Any rash or fever after a tick bite should cause a prompt visit to the doctor.

Other Insect Bites

Most other insect bites and spider bites result in pain, swelling, and/or redness. There's discomfort, but usually no reason for serious worry. Bites from insects which are poisonous are most serious to the very young, the very old, and people with serious underlying medical problems.

1. If you can do it safely, try to capture or at least identify the insect – killing it is ok, if necessary, but try not to crush it beyond recognition.

2. If the bite is from a black widow or brown recluse spider, **get medical attention promptly.**

3. Clean the wound with soap and water. Use a disinfectant if available.

4. Monitor the victim for any signs of infection or disease. If the pain does not diminish in 48 hours, get medical attention.

Snake and Animal Bites

Snake Bites

The vast majority of snake bites are by non-poisonous snakes, and even bites from poisonous snakes do not result in envenomation about 25% of the time. Of the approximately 8,000 bites annually by poisonous snakes, only 10-12 are fatal.

- **Don't use tourniquets, make incisions, apply suction, or apply electrical current to snake-bites.**

1. Check the victims ABCs. If you need to, begin rescue breathing and/or CPR **(see CPR pages 71-74)**. Get medical help.

2. Watch for signs of shock and treat for shock if necessary **(see Shock page 81)**.

3. If you can do it safely, try to identify the snake.

4. Try to keep the victim calm and inactive.

5. Stop bleeding by applying direct pressure.

6. Keep the affected part of the body below the level of the heart.

7. Apply a sterile dressing and bandage **(see Cleaning and Bandaging Wounds page 78)**.

8. Get prompt medical attention.

Animal Bites
For all animal bites, seek medical attention promptly.

1. Check the victims ABCs. If you need to, begin rescue breathing and/or CPR **(see CPR pages 71-74)**. Get medical help.

2. Watch for signs of shock and treat for shock if necessary **(see Shock page 81)**.

3. Try to keep the victim calm.

4. Stop bleeding by applying direct pressure and elevating the wound above the level of the heart **(see Bleeding pages 75-76)**.

5. Apply a sterile dressing and bandage **(see Cleaning and Bandaging Wounds page 78)**.

6. Get prompt medical attention.

Bone and Joint Injuries

Dislocated and broken bones are common injuries that range from minor to very serious. In either case, you should get medical help. Giving the proper first aid may not only ease the amount of immediate suffering, but also may lessen the ultimate severity of the injury. A fracture should be suspected if a deformity is present, the victim is unable to move the injured part, or the victim reports that they heard a "snap" or cracking noise. Fractures or joint injuries typically result in severe pain and swelling, and may have bluish discoloration and/or numbness or tingling sensation below the injury site.

EMS If there is severe bleeding associated with a dislocated or broken bone, apply direct pressure (see Bleeding pages 75-76) and call EMS.

EMS If you can't immobilize the injury yourself, call EMS before moving the victim.

EMS If the victim has a broken hip, pelvis or upper leg, do not move the victim. Call EMS.

- **Don't move the victim unless the injury is immobilized.**

- **Don't change the position of a misshapen bone or joint.**

- **Don't give the victim anything to eat or drink.**

1. Check the victims ABCs. If you need to, begin rescue breathing and/or CPR **(see CPR pages 71-74)**. Get medical help.

2. Try to keep the victim calm and still.

3. If the skin is pierced by a broken bone, it is important that you give first aid to prevent infection and control the bleeding **(see Bleeding pages 75-76)**.

4. Immobilize the injured area with a splint or sling. The specific type of splint or sling used depends on the location of the injury. See the following pages for various types of splints and slings and their applications.

5. Cover the victim with a blanket or anything handy that will keep the victim warm and prevent shock **(see Shock page 81)**.

6. Give first aid for other injuries.

7. Get medical help or stay with the victim until medical help arrives.

Splints

(Lower Leg, Knee, Ankle, Finger, Toe, Ribs)
A splint is used to immobilize an injured area until you have medical help. Be sure to give first aid to wounds before you apply a splint. Splints can be made from just about anything (boards, sticks, umbrellas) that will give strong, straight support. A splint should be much longer than the bone that is broken – it should prevent movement of the joints above and below the fracture **(see illustration 15)**. Pieces of cloth can be used to secure the splint to the injured limb. The ties should be tight enough that they are secure, but loose enough so they don't cut off circulation.

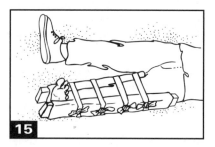

15

Lower Leg

Two padded boards work best as splints for leg injuries. One board on the outside of the injured leg (from the hip to just beyond the foot), and the other board on the inside of the injured leg (from the groin to just beyond the foot). Tie the splint in at least four places. If you don't have boards, place pillows or a blanket between the victims legs and tie both legs together with cloth ties **(see illustration 16)**.

Knee

An injured knee that's in a straight position should be treated the same way you would treat an injured leg (above). If the knee is bent, don't straighten it. Simply bend the uninjured leg so that it matches the position of the injured leg. Then place pillows or a blanket between the legs and tie both legs together with cloth ties **(see illustration 17)**.

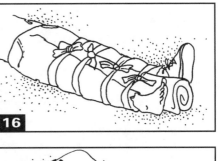

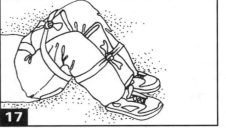

Ankle

Immobilize the ankle by folding a blanket or pillow around the base of the foot and ankle and tie it in several places. Leave the toes showing **(see illustration 18)**. Elevate the lower leg and apply a cold compress if available.

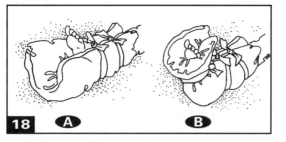

18 Ⓐ Ⓑ

Finger or Toe

A broken finger or toe usually doesn't require medical attention unless it is misshapen. The injured digit can be taped to an adjacent finger or toe with a piece of gauze or cotton placed between them. Apply a cold compress and elevate the injured extremity.

Ribs

Support the injured side with a pillow and get medical help. If necessary, give first aid for breathing problems **(see Breathing Problems page 98)**.

Slings

(Arm and Collarbone, Elbow, Wrist)

A sling is used to support and immobilize shoulder, collar bone and arm injuries. A broken arm, for example, would require a splint first, and then a sling. You can make a sling from any large piece of cloth, even a shirt or sweater will do. The material you make the sling from should be folded into a triangle with the base of the triangle about 55 inches long and the sides about 40 inches long .

Arm and Collarbone

Carefully slide the sling under the injured arm with the point of the triangle under the elbow. Leave the fingers exposed. Tie the sling on the opposite side of the victim's neck. Fold over the extra cloth at the victim's elbow and secure it with safety pins or tie it in a knot. Be sure the sling is tight enough to provide support, yet loose enough to be comfortable **(see illustration 19)**.

Elbow

If the arm is bent at the elbow, apply a sling as you would for an arm or collarbone. If the arm is not bent, do not force it into a sling.

Wrist

For an injured wrist, apply a sling as you would for an arm or collarbone but first pad the wrist well by wrapping it with a towel or magazine.

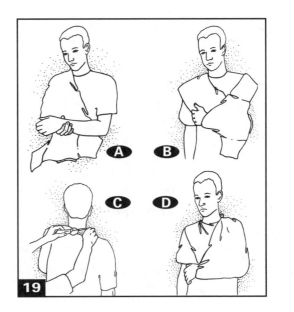

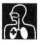

Breathing Problems

Breathing problems can occur for a variety of reasons, including sudden illness or injury, allergic reaction, choking, drug abuse, heart attack or poisoning, as well as health problems like heart disease, emphysema and asthma. Try to discover the cause of the breathing problem and treat it accordingly.

Since breathing is essential to life, and since we do it constantly and automatically, a sudden problem with breathing can be very frightening. It's important that first aid should include a calm, relaxed demeanor on the part of the first aid giver.

EMS **If the victim is experiencing breathing problems, call EMS.**

- **Don't support the victim's head with a pillow.**

1. Check the victims ABCs. If you need to, begin rescue breathing and/or CPR **(see CPR pages 71-74)**. Get medical help.

2. Let the patient sit or lay in a position which is comfortable for them – usually, sitting up makes breathing a bit easier.

3. Loosen clothing and/or jewelry that may restrict breathing and circulation.

4. Care for any neck or chest wounds **(see Bleeding page 75, and Cleaning and Bandaging Wounds page 78)**.

5. If the victim's chest moves in a lop-sided manner while attempting to breathe, ribs may be broken. Use a pillow to give support to the injured side and get medical help.

6. If home oxygen is available, provide oxygen using the delivery system available to the victim.

7. Monitor the victim's ABCs until medical help arrives.

Burns

Burns can be superficial or severe, but regardless of the degree, they are almost always extremely painful. The amount of suffering can be lessened greatly if the proper first aid is given prior to seeking medical attention.

For All Burns:

- **Don't allow the burn to become contaminated. Keeping the burned area as clean as possible is important.**

- **Don't break blisters or touch the burned area.**

- **Don't apply ointment, cream, oil, spray, or any household remedy.**

- **Don't apply ice directly to the skin.**

Severe Burns

Burns are severe if they involve the hands, feet, genitalia, neck, or face; if they were caused by electricity or chemicals; if the victim is experiencing any difficulty breathing or has underlying medical problems; if any burn more significant than a sunburn covers an area of the body which is greater than the size of the victim's chest; or if the burned areas are hard and black, grey, or white ("full-thickness"). **Always call EMS or get medical attention immediately for severe burns.**

EMS **If you think a burn is severe (or you're not sure), call EMS.**

- **Don't apply cold water or ice to a severe burn.**

1. Check the victims ABCs. If you need to, begin rescue breathing and/or CPR **(see CPR pages 71-74)**. Get medical help.

2. Carefully remove any clothing or jewelry from the burned area, if you can do so easily.

3. Cover the wound with a dry, sterile dressing. Don't use cotton or adhesive tape.

4. If possible, keep the burned area elevated above the level of the heart. Protect it from pressure and friction.

5. Take steps to prevent shock **(see Shock page 81).**

6. Continue to monitor the victim's ABCs until medical help arrives.

Superficial Burns

Symptoms include pain, redness, swelling and blistering.

EMS If a burn covers a large area, even if it's superficial, call EMS or seek medical help.

• **Don't apply cold water if the burn is larger than the victim's chest. Get medical help.**

1. Keep the victim calm.

2. Carefully remove any clothing or jewelry from the burned area, if you can do so easily.

3. Cool the burned area by holding it under cold running water if possible, or by continuously applying clean, cold wet cloths.

4. Cover the burned area with a clean, dry dressing. Don't use anything that will stick to the burned area.

5. If possible, keep the burned area elevated above the level of the heart. Protect it from pressure and friction.

6. If signs of infection develop, which include increased pain, redness, swelling and discharge, get medical help.

Choking

Breathing difficulties are serious and can be quite frightening for the victim. Choking is especially serious since it can happen very quickly and can be immediately life threatening. It occurs most often in adults who eat while intoxicated or who do not properly chew or cut their food, and in children while running or playing with food in their mouths. Common signs that a person is choking include anxiously holding the throat; an inability to speak; weak, ineffective coughing; and pale or blue coloration of the skin, especially of the face.

EMS If the victim is obviously choking and can't speak, call EMS.

• **Don't give first aid if the victim is able to breathe through their mouth and/or coughing. Stay with the victim and be ready to give first aid if the victim's condition gets worse.**

1. When the victim is unable to breathe and has shown signs of choking, or rescue breathing seems to be obstructed, prepare to do the Heimlich (abdominal thrust) maneuver **(see illustration 20)**. Position yourself behind the victim with your arms around the victim's stomach. If the victim is too large for you to get your arms around, **see Chest Thrusts on the next page.**

2. Place the thumb-side of your fist above the victim's navel and below the lower end of the breastbone.

3. Take hold of your fist with your free hand.

4. Pull your fist upward and in quickly and firmly. This should force air out of the windpipe and pop out the object that's choking the victim. Continue with thrusts until the airway is clear.

5. If the object is removed through this procedure, it is important that the victim still receive medical attention, since complications may arise.

Chest Thrusts

If the victim is too large for you to get your arms around (e.g. obese or pregnant), give chest thrusts in place of abdominal thrusts **(see illustration 21)**.

1. From behind the choking victim (the victim may be sitting or standing), put your arms under the armpits with thumb-side of your fist in the center of the victim's breastbone (not on the ribs).

2 Take hold of your fist with your free hand.

3. Pull your fist toward the victim's backbone. This should force air out of the windpipe and remove the object that's choking the victim. Continue with thrusts until the airway is clear.

4. If the object is removed through this procedure, it is important that the victim still receives medical attention, since complications may arise.

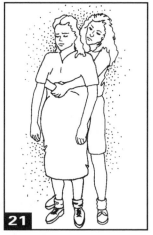

Cold Exposure

Frostbite occurs when areas of skin and underlying tissue freeze; hypothermia occurs when the whole body cools down. You don't have to live in an area that experiences harsh winter months to encounter either frostbite or hypothermia. In both cases, the symptoms may start out slowly, but can worsen quickly, and hypothermia may become life-threatening if first aid is not implemented quickly.

Frostbite

Exposed skin (ears and nose) and areas with poor blood flow (i.e., toes and feet if boots are too tight) are at greatest risk.

The signs and symptoms of frostbite include skin that's red and painful in the early stages and white and numb in the late stages. Severe frostbite may result in blisters, gangrene, and hard, frozen skin.

EMS **If the victim has both frostbite and hypothermia, call EMS and then give first aid for the hypothermia.**

EMS **If the victim has frostbite in the later stages, call EMS.**

- **Don't rub or massage frostbitten areas.**

- **Don't apply hot water or strong, direct heat.**

- **Don't warm a frostbitten area if you can't keep it warm thereafter.**

- **Don't let the victim drink alcohol or smoke cigarettes – both contribute to poor circulation.**

1. Get the victim out of the cold and into a warm place.

2. Gently remove any jewelry or clothing that restricts circulation.

3. Warm the frostbitten areas by either placing them in warm water or covering them with warm towels until the skin is soft, becomes flushed (bright red) and sensation returns – this may take more than 30 minutes in some cases.

4. As frostbitten areas are rewarmed, they can become very painful. Try to keep the victim calm.

5. Apply clean, dry dressings to rewarmed frostbitten areas. Also, use dressings to keep frostbitten toes and fingers slightly separated.

Hypothermia

Hypothermia occurs when a victim's body temperature drops below normal; it is caused by exposure to cool or cold (but not necessarily freezing) temperatures. The elderly, infants, people with lower percentages of body fat, and alcoholics are more susceptible to hypothermia, but anyone can become hypothermic if they are exposed to low temperatures for an extended period of time. Symptoms of mild hypothermia may include shivering, loss of coordination, or some confusion. Victims of severe hypothermia typically can no longer shiver, and they may experience generalized weakness, muscle stiffness, an irregular and/or slow heart beat, confusion and unconsciousness.

EMS **If the victim has severe hypothermia, call EMS before you give first aid.**

EMS **If the victim has only mild hypothermia, give first aid and then get medical help.**

EMS **If the victim has hypothermia and frostbite, call EMS, then give first aid for the hypothermia.**

- **Don't assume that above-freezing temperatures will prevent hypothermia, and remember that if the victim is already hypothermic, any cool environment will continue to make them worse, even if you are comfortable.**

- **Don't apply hot water or strong, direct heat.**

- **Don't warm a mildly hypothermic victim if you can't keep the victim warm.**

- **Don't let the victim drink alcohol or smoke cigarettes, both contribute to poor circulation.**

1. Check the victims ABCs. If you need to, begin rescue breathing and/or CPR **(see CPR pages 71-74).** Get medical help.

2. Move a severe hypothermia victim gently – low body temperature puts people at a higher risk of heart attack.

3. Try to assure that the victim doesn't get any colder. Bring the victim indoors, if possible, and remove any wet or restrictive clothing.

4. Apply warm compresses to the neck, chest, underarm, and groin area. If necessary, rewarm the victim with your own body heat through skin-to-skin contact. Cover the victim with a blanket to prevent further heat loss (but remember that this will not warm them). Ensure that the head and neck are also covered **(see illustration 22).**

5. If the victim is alert and can easily swallow, give the victim warm, sweetened liquids or soup.

6. Stay with the victim until medical help arrives.

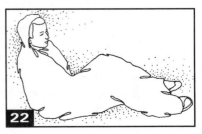

22

Drowning

Anyone can drown, regardless of age or swimming ability. Drowning deaths are caused by lack of oxygen, which is known as asphyxiation. A drowning victim may or may not be breathing when rescued, depending upon the stage at which the victim is found. The victim may have a bluish face, especially the lips and ears, or may be pale in appearance.

Ensure your own safety first! In their panic, a drowning person will climb on top of you, pushing you under water. It is safer to reach to them with something, or throw something they can grab, rather than going out into the water, even if you can swim well.

EMS Before performing any first aid procedures, other than removing the victim from the water, call EMS (if more than one person is present, EMS should be called while rescue is taking place).

EMS Even after a victim is revived, medical help should be sought since lung and other complications may occur later.

- Don't give a victim of near-drowning alcohol or cigarettes.

1. Remove the drowning victim from the water to a safe place (i.e., above high tide) if you can do so without putting your own life at risk.

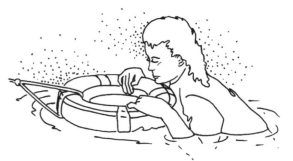

2. Check the victims ABCs **(see CPR page 72).** If you need to, begin rescue breathing and/or CPR. If the victim's ABCs are present and you don't suspect a spinal injury, place the victim in the recovery position **(see Unconsciousness page 85).**

3. Remove wet clothes and cover the victim with a blanket or anything handy that will keep them warm.

4. Watch for signs of hypothermia **(see Hypothermia on pages 104-105).**

5. Give first aid for other injuries.

6. Stay with the victim until medical help arrives.

Eye Injury

Eye injuries can be devastating and lead to loss of vision, so proper first aid may help prevent blindness. The most common eye injuries include having something (a foreign body) "stuck" in the eye, and cuts or blows (trauma) to the eye. Also, eyes may come in contact with chemicals **(see Poison and Chemical Exposure page 119)**. The best thing to do in most eye injury cases is to seek medical help promptly.

Something Stuck in the Eye

EMS **If the injury is a result of high-speed fragments (i.e., from a grinder), if blood is seen on or around the eye, if the victim cannot see clearly, or if there is severe pain, call EMS.**

EMS **If an object is impaled in the eye, call EMS. Do not remove the impaled object!**

- **Don't rub or press on the injured eye – this can embed the foreign body or aggravate the injury further.**

- **Don't use cotton or sharp objects like a tweezers to aid in removing something from the eye.**

1. If an impaled object is seen, it should be left in place and protected against further movement by covering with a cup **(see illustration 23)**. **Call EMS.**

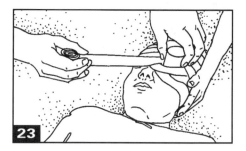

2. If there is not an object impaled in the eye, move the victim to a well-lit area. Conduct a thorough search for the object by having the victim slowly move the eye in all directions. Check the inside of the victim's upper and lower eyelid, since foreign bodies frequently lodge there **(see illustration 24)**.

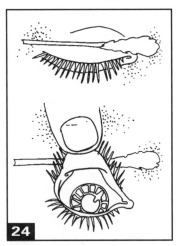

3. If you locate the object on the inner surface of the eyelid or resting on the eye itself, flush it out with a steady stream of fresh water or gently lift it off with a clean cloth **(see illustration 25)**. Sharp objects like tweezers and toothpicks should not be used.

4. If you can't remove the object or it appears embedded, get medical help immediately. It's best to gently cover both eyes with clean, dry dressings to reduce eye movement. Talk with the victim after the eyes are patched to help keep them calm.

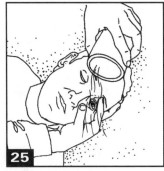

5. If the victim experiences pain in the eye, or has trouble seeing clearly with the eye after the object has been removed, get medical help.

Trauma (cuts or blows) to the Eye

EMS **If the injury is a result of significant force (i.e., from a motor vehicle accident), if blood is seen on or around the eye, if the victim cannot see clearly, or if there is severe pain, call EMS.**

• **Don't rub or press on the injured eye.**

• **Don't use raw steak or an ice pack on an injured eye.**

1. If the eye appears cut, do not apply pressure. Gently cover with a sterile dressing and seek medical attention immediately.

2. If a "black eye" is developing, gently apply cold compresses (a towel soaked in cold water or wrapped around a bag of ice) to reduce the pain and swelling, and to help stop any bleeding. Keep the victim's head elevated to reduce the swelling and pain.

3. If bleeding continues, if the patient complains of problems with vision, or if you think the eye may be damaged, get medical help.

Head, Face and Nose Injuries

Head injuries include any blow or trauma to the head as well as face, mouth and nose injuries. With injuries to any of these areas, the first aid giver should also suspect spinal injury. Head injuries are serious if the patient is (or has been) unconscious, is confused, vomits, is having (or has had) a seizure, has different-sized pupils, is partially paralyzed, or complains of tingling in extremities. Symptoms of spinal injury include back and/or neck pain, numbness, tingling, and loss of feeling in the arms and/or legs. If these symptoms are present, or if you simply suspect spinal injury, give first aid for spinal injury **(see Spinal Injury page 83)**.

Head Injuries

EMS If you think the head injury is serious (or your aren't sure), call EMS.

- **Don't move the victim unless absolutely necessary.**

- **Don't remove any object from the wound.**

1. Check the victims ABCs. If you need to, begin rescue breathing and/or CPR **(see CPR pages 71-74)**. Get medical help.

2. If the victim is unconscious, assume the victim has suffered a spinal injury and give first aid accordingly **(see Spinal Injury page 83)**. If the victim is conscious, make sure the victim remains as still as possible.

3. If the victim has seizures, **see Seizures page 123**.

4. For bleeding wounds, don't apply direct pressure if you think the victim may have a skull fracture. Bandage the wound firmly but without applying pressure directly over the suspected fracture area, and get medical help immediately.

5. For superficial wounds in which you don't suspect a skull fracture, apply direct pressure, then bandage the wound and get medical help. A briskly bleeding scalp wound may cause the patient to lose a great deal of blood, resulting in shock.

6. Apply a cold compress (a towel soaked in cold water or wrapped around a bag of ice) to swelling areas.

7. Even if the injury is minor, it's important that the victim see a doctor since complications may arise over time, especially if there was any period of unconsciousness or if the victim does not remember the incident.

Face Injuries

EMS If you think the face injury is serious, or if there's any difficulty breathing, call EMS.

- **Don't forget the possibility of head, neck or spinal injury.**

- **Don't give the victim anything to eat or drink.**

- **Don't attempt to adjust broken facial bones.**

1. Check the victim's ABCs **(see CPR page 72)**. If necessary begin rescue breathing and/or CPR and get medical help. Jaw and mouth injuries make it difficult to perform traditional rescue breathing, so you may need to use mouth-to-nose breathing instead of mouth-to-mouth.

2. If the victim is unconscious, assume the victim has suffered a spinal injury and give first aid accordingly **(see Spinal Injury page 83)**. If the victim is conscious, make sure the victim remains as still as possible.

3. If you don't suspect a spinal injury, place the victim in the recovery position **(see Unconsciousness page 85)**.

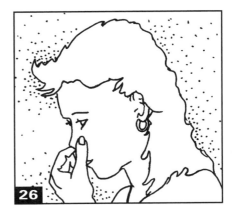

4. Control bleeding by applying direct pressure. If you suspect broken or fractured facial bones, apply the direct pressure gently.

Nosebleeds

EMS **If you think the bleeding or the injury that caused it is serious, call EMS.**

1. Keep the victim calm.

2. Have the victim breathe through his or her mouth.

3. Have the victim sit down and lean forward, not backward. Leaning forward will prevent blood from draining in the victim's throat.

4. While the victim is leaning forward, firmly pinch the soft part of the nose just under the bony ridge for 15 to 20 minutes **(see illustration 26).**

5. Place a cold compress (a towel soaked in cold water or wrapped around a bag of ice) on the bridge of the nose to reduce swelling.

6. If bleeding continues, repeat steps 3, 4 and 5 above. If bleeding persists, get medical help.

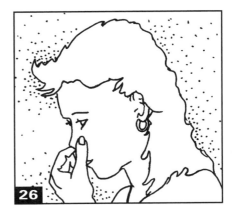

26

Broken Nose

EMS **If you think the nose is broken, get medical help. If you think the injury is serious, or if you suspect head, neck or spinal injury, call EMS.**

- **Don't try to adjust broken facial bones.**

1. Keep the victim calm.

2. Encourage the victim to breathe through the mouth.

3. Make the victim sit down and lean forward, not backward. Leaning forward will prevent blood from draining in the victim's throat.

4. Apply a cold compress to the nose (the victim will know how much pressure to apply) until you have medical help.

Heart Attack

A heart attack occurs when heart muscle gets less oxygen than it needs – either because the arteries going to the heart are blocked or because the arteries go into spasm. Factors which put someone especially at risk for heart attacks include being male, advancing age, smoking, high blood pressure, being overweight, having a high cholesterol level (a diet with too much fat), having diabetes, getting too little exercise, and the use of "stimulant" drugs.

Common symptoms include: pressure or pain in the middle of the chest (under the breastbone) which may radiate up into the neck and jaw, to between the shoulder blades, or down the left arm; shortness of breath; heart palpitations; sweating; dizziness; and pale skin. Sometimes, the sensation of indigestion occurs instead of the chest pain. Symptoms can be quite variable and at times only one of these symptoms will occur.

EMS If you suspect a person is experiencing a heart attack, call EMS.

- **Don't wait to see if the victim's condition improves.**

- **Don't give the victim anything by mouth, unless it's a prescription drug which has been ordered specifically for the victim's heart condition (i.e., a nitroglycerin tablet).**

1. Check the victim's ABCs **(see CPR page 72)**. If you need to, begin rescue breathing and/or CPR.

2. Stay with the victim until medical help arrives. If the victim loses consciousness, check the victim's ABCs and give first aid for an unconscious victim **(see Unconsciousness page 85)**.

3. Make the victim as calm and as comfortable as possible. Loosen any tight clothing. Reassure the victim that help is on the way.

4. If home oxygen is available, provide oxygen using the delivery system available to the victim.

The body's temperature can be raised in a number of ways including a hot outside temperature (especially with high humidity), poor ventilation, exercise, sudden illness, some medications, and as a result of pre-existing medical conditions.

Heat stroke occurs when the body's temperature rises above 106° Fahrenheit. Heat stroke is a true medical emergency! Its symptoms include dry, hot and red skin; rapid and weak pulse; rapid, shallow breathing; confusion; weakness, seizures and unconsciousness.

Heat exhaustion is an intermediate and generalized form of heat illness. Its symptoms vary, but may include weakness, light-headedness, nausea, vomiting, and headache. As symptoms become more severe, the victim may develop a rapid heart rate, rapid breathing rate, and/or become unconscious.

Heat cramps are the least severe form of heat illness, usually associated with strenuous exercise. Victims experience painful spasms of their muscles and frequently sweat profusely.

Heat Stroke

EMS **If you suspect heat stroke, call EMS.**

Don't give the victim anything by mouth, including salted drinks, salt tablets, or any other medications unless told to do so by medical professional.

1. Keep the victim cool while you wait for EMS to arrive. Move the victim to a cooler environment. Administer cold compresses to the victim's neck, groin and armpits. Gently spray the victim with cool water. Fan the victim if possible.

2. Monitor the victim for signs of shock **(see Shock page 81).**

3. If the victim has seizures, give first aid for seizures **(see Seizures page 123)**.

4. If the victim loses consciousness, give first aid for unconsciousness **(see Unconsciousness page 85)**.

Heat Exhaustion and Heat Cramps

EMS **If symptoms do not resolve promptly, call EMS.**

- **Don't let the victim drink alcohol or caffeine.**

- **Don't give the victim aspirin or other over-the-counter medications to reduce fever.**

- **Don't give the victim salt tablets.**

1. Encourage the victim to lay down and rest.

2. Keep the victim cool by moving the victim to a cooler environment. Administer cold compresses to the victim's neck, groin and armpits. Fan the victim if possible.

3. If the victim is fully alert, give the victim salt-containing beverages to sip (like Gatorade® or a similar sports beverage), or make a slightly salty drink by mixing 1 teaspoon of salt to 1 quart of water.

4. Monitor the victim for signs of shock **(see Shock page 81)**.

5. If the victim has seizures, give first aid for seizures **(see Seizures page 123)**.

6. If the victim loses consciousness, give first aid for unconsciousness **(see Unconsciousness page 85)**.

Muscle Injuries

A muscle cramp occurs when a muscle suddenly becomes tight. Cramps can happen when muscles are working or when they're resting, and can be caused by medications or dehydration. A strained (pulled) muscle occurs when muscle fibers are damaged or torn; a sprain happens when the bands (ligaments) between bones at joints are stretched or torn. Signs and symptoms of sprains and strains include pain or tenderness at the joint (or just above or below), swelling, and/or black and blue discoloration.

Muscle Cramps

- **Don't ever apply heat directly to the skin.**

1. Have the victim slowly and gently stretch the cramped muscle.

2. Apply a warm, moist cloth or a heating pad covered by a towel to the muscle.

3. If cramps continue, get medical attention.

Strains & Sprains

EMS **If the victim is experiencing severe pain, or if you think a bone may have been broken, call EMS or get professional medical assistance.**

- **Don't ever apply ice directly to the skin.**

1. Remove any clothing or jewelry that may restrict circulation in the affected extremity.

2. Keep the muscle rested and elevated, if possible, for at least 24 hours.

3. Apply cold compresses for about 20 minutes every few hours for the first 24 hours; then apply moist, warm compresses for about 20 minutes several times each day for several days thereafter.

Poison and Chemical Exposure

Aperson may come in contact with poison by eating (ingesting) or breathing (inhaling) a poisonous substance, or by a spill to the skin or a splash to the eye. Symptoms of poison exposure vary depending upon the type of poison, the health, the size (weight and age) of the victim, and the time elapsed since exposure. Signs and symptoms can appear as quickly as several minutes after exposure, or may not appear until several hours after exposure. When you know that an exposure has taken place, don't wait for symptoms to appear before taking action.

Parents of young children must assume a poisoning has taken place if they find a pill bottle or other container out of place or in a child's possession; if a there is evidence that a child has eaten wild berries, mushrooms or flowers; if a child's breath smells of chemicals; or if there are signs of the poison around the child's mouth.

The first aid you give before you get medical help can reduce the seriousness of the poisoning, and in some cases, prevent the need for hospitalization.

Poison Ingestion

- **Don't induce vomiting unless a medical professional instructs you to do so.**

- **Don't try to neutralize the chemical without consulting your local Poison Control Center or physician (even if the instructions on the product label tell you to do so).**

- **Don't give the victim anything to eat or drink if the victim is drowsy, unconscious, having a seizure, or is having trouble swallowing.**

- **Don't assume that product label information is correct.**

1. Remove any poison substance from the victim's mouth.

2. Check the victims ABCs. If you need to, begin rescue breathing and/or CPR **(see CPR pages 71-74).** Get medical help.

3. Give a few sips of milk or water if the victim is awake and able to swallow.

4. Try to specifically identify what caused the poisoning.

5. Call your local Poison Control Center. If you don't have one in your area, or can't find the number quickly, call EMS.

6. If the victim is having seizures, give first aid for seizures **(see Seizures page 123).**

7. Collect all containers for review and a sample of the poison substance in case it needs to be analyzed.

8. Keep the victim calm and relaxed while you wait for medical help.

Poison Inhalation

- **Don't give the victim anything to eat or drink if the victim is drowsy, unconscious, having a seizures or is having trouble swallowing.**

- **Don't assume that product label information is correct.**

- **Don't enter an area contaminated by poison (carbon monoxide, chlorine, natural gas etc.) Call EMS.**

1. Get the victim out of the contaminated area. Open windows to help fresh air circulate.

2. Check the victims ABCs. If you need to, begin rescue breathing and/or CPR **(see CPR pages 71-74).** Get medical help.

3. Call your local Poison Control Center. If you don't have one in your area, or can't find the number quickly, call EMS.

4. If the victim is having seizures, give first aid for seizures **(see Seizures page 123).**

5. Try to keep the victim calm and relaxed while you wait for medical help.

Skin Exposure to Chemicals

- **Don't touch the exposed area.**

- **Don't try to neutralize the chemical. Consult your local Poison Control Center or physician.**

- **Don't apply anything to the exposed area, including creams, oils or sprays.**

- **Don't break blisters.**

1. Remove any contaminated clothing from the victim and flush the contaminated skin area with fresh water and mild soap for 20 minutes. Be careful not to contaminate yourself.

2. Call your local Poison Control Center. If you don't have one in your area, or can't find the number quickly, call EMS.

3. Try to identify the chemical.

4. After flushing the area thoroughly, apply a cool, wet cloth to the area if the contaminated area is painful; otherwise, cover the area with a clean, dry dressing.

5. Keep the victim calm and relaxed while you wait for medical help.

Skin Exposure to Poison Ivy, Poison Oak, or Poison Sumac

- **Don't burn these plants – they produce toxic fumes which may result in a life-threatening reaction.**

1. Wash the irritated skin area thoroughly with fresh water and mild soap. Wash the contaminated clothing.

2. If the area becomes infected, or does not improve after several days, seek medical attention.

Eye Exposure

The importance of early and aggressive irrigation at the scene cannot be over-emphasized. All chemical exposures to the eyes mandate medical attention.

- **Don't flush chemicals from one eye into the other – pour fluids into the eye from the side**

closest to the nose, and let the water run out the side closest to the ear (see illustration 27).

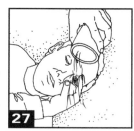

1. Gently flush the eye with luke-warm water for 20 minutes. This is best done by leaning the victim over a sink and pouring water across the eye, or by having the victim stand in a shower and letting the water strike the forehead and nose and flow across the eye.

2. Call your local Poison Control Center. If you don't have one in your area, or can't find the number quickly, call EMS.

3. Try to specifically identify what caused the poisoning.

4. Keep the eyes closed or apply a cold cloth over the eyes. Get the victim medical attention immediately.

Seizures

Seizures happen when muscles suddenly and involuntarily contract. There's nothing you can do as a first aid giver to stop someone from having seizures. But there's much you can do to see that they don't harm themselves while they're seizing.

EMS Call EMS if the victim:

- has a seizure that lasts longer than 2 minutes,
- has more than 1 seizure in an hour,
- doesn't wake up completely between seizures,
- has never had seizures before (or if you are unsure),
- has diabetes, high blood pressure, or is pregnant,
- had the seizure in the water (i.e., a pool, lake)

- **Don't restrain the victim or attempt any first aid while the victim is having a seizure.**
- **Don't move the victim unless you need to get the victim away from danger.**
- **Don't attempt to put anything in the victim's mouth during a seizure.**

1. If you are present when the victim feels a seizure coming on, help the victim lie down in a safe place (like the floor), away from furniture and stairs, etc. If possible, try to cushion the area with soft things like pillows, blankets or clothing.

2. Loosen any tight clothing, especially around the victim's neck.

3. Allow the victim to seize – don't interfere with the victim's movements.

4. After the seizure, if you don't think the victim has suffered a spinal injury, place the victim in the recovery position **(see Unconsciousness page 85).**

5. If the victim vomits, and you have no reason to suspect a spinal injury, put the victim in the recovery position quickly, and sweep the mouth out with a cloth or napkin. If the victim may have a spinal injury and is vomiting or choking on fluids, slowly and gently roll the victim onto his or her side, keeping the victim's head, neck and back supported and in-line. And again, if you have to move the victim, do so with the help of people around you.

6. Check the victim's ABCs **(see CPR page 72)** and watch for signs of more seizures.

7. After the seizure has passed, the victim will usually be confused and/or sleepy. Let them rest quietly.

8. Stay with the victim until fully recovered or until medical help arrives. Do not allow them to drive a car for several hours after the seizure.

Stroke

A stroke is caused when a blood vessel in the brain bursts or becomes narrowed by a clot. Recognizing the signs of stroke and getting medical help immediately can greatly improve the victim's chances for recovery.

Signs and symptoms of a stroke include sudden confusion, dizziness, severe headache, sudden onset of weakness in the face, arm or leg on one side of the body, a loss of speech or difficulty speaking, new vision problems and unconsciousness.

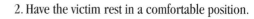 **If you suspect the victim has suffered a stroke, call EMS.**

• **Don't give the victim anything to eat or drink.**

1. Check the victims ABCs **(see CPR page 72)**. If necessary, begin rescue breathing and/or CPR. Get medical help immediately.

2. Have the victim rest in a comfortable position.

3. If the victim loses consciousness, place the victim in the recovery position **(see Unconsciousness page 85)**.

4. Continue to monitor the victim's ABCs until medical help arrives.

125

Index

(Also see Survival supplies checklists)

Survival supplies checklists, 9-13
    automobile,13
    clothing, 9
    first aid, See First aid supplies checklist
    food and water, 10
    hygiene, 11
    miscellaneous supplies, 12
    tools, 11

Sweating, as a symptom associated with:
    heart attack, 115
    heat illness, 23,116

Swelling, as a sign or symptom associated with:
    allergic reaction, 87
    bite or sting, 89-91
    bone and joint injuries, 93
    burns, 100
    facial injuries, 112
    eye injuries, 110
    head injuries, 111-112
    internal bleeding (abdominal), 77
    muscle injuries, 118
    nose injuries, 113

T

Tags, bracelets, See Medical Alert tags

Temperature, body, as associated with:
    heat illness, 23,116
    hypothermia, 25, 104-105
    shock, 81
    tick bites, 91

Tetanus immunization, See Cleaning and Bandaging Wounds

Tick bites, See Bites and Stings

Tidal Waves (tsunamis), See Earthquakes

Tingling, See Numbness or tingling as a symptom

Toe injuries, See Bone and Joint Injuries; Cold Exposure (frostbite)

Tools, See Survival Supplies checklists

Tornadoes, 46-48
    shelter in your home, 47
    shelter outside, 48
    survival supplies, See Survival Supplies
    watches and warnings, 46-47

U

Unconsciousness, 85-86
    checking for consciousness, 85-86
    first aid for, 85-86
    recovery position for, 86
    when to use recovery position:
    near-drowning, 107
    head or facial injury, 112
    seizures, 124
    stroke, 125

Unconsciousness as a symptom associated with:
    allergic reaction, 87-88
    near-drowning, 107
    head injuries, 112
    hypothermia, 23, 104
    heart attack, 115
    heat illness, 116-117
    poison or chemical exposure, 119-120
    seizures, 124
    stroke, 125

Urine, blood in, as a sign of:
    internal bleeding, 77

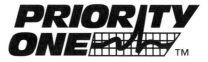

PRIORITY ONE™

Important Telephone Numbers

Personal Medical Profile Forms

Personal Property Profile Forms

Important Telephone Numbers

Emergency..**9-1-1**
In a life threatening emergency, dial 9-1-1 or your
local emergency medical services system number.

Our Telephone #

Our Address

Ambulance

Fire Department

Police

Poison Control Center

Hospital

Hospital Emergency Department

Name   /#
Family Physician

Name   /#
Family Physician

Gas Company

Electric Company

Name _____ /# _____
Neighbors

Name _____ /# _____
Neighbors

Name _____ /# _____
Baby Sitter

Name _____ /# _____
Friends

Name _____ /# _____
Friends

Family Work Numbers

Name _____ /# _____
Father

Name _____ /# _____
Mother

Name _____ /# _____
Other

Out-of-State Contact

Name _____

_____ / _____
City   **State**

_____ # _____
Telephone (Daytime)   **(Evening)**

Personal Medical Profile Form

(Make additional copies as needed)

Name
_____

Address
_____

City   / State   / Zip
_____

Height   / Weight   / Date Info Taken
_____

Birth Date   / Social Security Number
_____

Blood Type
_____

Family Physician   /# Phone
_____

Other Physician   /# Phone
_____

Insurance Co.   / Policy Number
_____

Contact   /# Phone
_____

Prescription Medications

_____

_____

_____

_____

Check any of the following medical conditions or problems that apply to the individual listed on the previous page. After each condition or problem checked, list any information you feel necessary (specific type or severity of problem etc.).

☐ **Allergies** _____

☐ **Asthma** _____

☐ **Bleeding Trait** _____

☐ **Concussion** _____

☐ **Diabetes/hypoglycemia** _____

☐ **Ear Problem** _____

☐ **Epilepsy** _____

☐ **Heart Problems** _____

☐ **High Blood Pressure** _____

☐ **Kidney Disorders** _____

☐ **Liver Disorders** _____

☐ **Mental Disorders** _____

☐ **Neurological Disorder** _____

☐ **Stroke/paralysis** _____

☐ **Thyroid Disorders** _____

☐ **Upper Respiratory Disorder** _____

☐ **Other** _____

_____

_____

Personal Property Profile Form

_____
Insurance Co.

_____
Policy Number

_____ /# _____
Contact   **Phone**

Check all of the following items that you own, noting the brand name, model and serial numbers when applicable.

☐ **Automobiles** _____

_____

_____

_____

☐ **Electronics (TVs, VCRs, video cameras)** _____

_____

_____

_____

_____

_____

☐ **Jewelry** _____

_____

_____

_____

☐ Collections (music, stamps, antiques, coins, art)

_____

_____

_____

_____

☐ Computer Equipment_____

_____

_____

_____

☐ Recreation Equipment (boats, jet skis, motorcy-cles, bicycles, camping equipment etc.) _____

_____

_____

_____

_____

_____

☐ Living Room Furniture _____

_____

☐ Dining Room Furniture _____

_____

☐ **Bedroom Furniture** _____

_____

☐ **Kitchen Furniture** _____

_____

☐ **Kitchen Appliances** _____

_____

_____

☐ **Clothing**_____

_____

_____

_____

☐ **Other**_____

_____

_____

_____

_____

_____

_____